The Other Awkward Age

The Other Awkward Age

Menopause

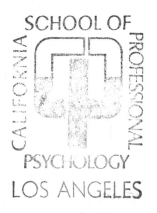

SCHOOL OF
CALIFORNIA PROFESSIONAL
PSYCHOLOGY
LOS ANGELES

Jane Page

TEN SPEED PRESS 1〰

Illustrated by Maryanne Hoburg

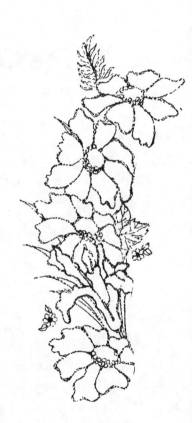

ISBN 0-913668-65-6 paper, $4.95
ISBN 0-913668-67-2 cloth, $8.95
Published by Ten Speed Press,
900 Modoc, Berkeley, Calif. 94707
Printed in the United States of America

I want to thank

all the women who have contributed to this book
by writing and talking to us at WOMEN IN MIDSTREAM,
University of Washington YWCA, with special thanks
to Irma Levine, Julie Campbell, and Virginia Scofield.
I would never have made it without their help.

I also extend special thanks to:
Professor Elaine Smith for commenting on our
discussion of sexuality;
Barbara Schneidman, M.D., for checking the manuscript
for medical accuracy;
Zola Ross and her writing group at the Women's
University Club for their helpful criticisms;
Verna Pedrin and Beverly Rutzick of the San Francisco
Women's Health Center for encouraging me when
I needed it most;
Drs. Donald C. Smith and Noel S. Weiss for permission
to quote from their interviews;
All the doctors who generously gave us their time
for interviews;
The American Cancer Society for permission to quote
their instructions for breast self-examination;
Ruby Apsler for her conscientious editorial work;
and my family and friends for bearing with me
during the nervous times.

Contents

Introduction
Why Write A Book About Menopause?

*How marvelous to find a group helping
the 'older' woman. We're all prepared
for menstruation, but we know so little about
menopause.*
From a letter to *Women in Midstream*

This book results from the efforts of many women: the group at the University of Washington WYCA in Seattle, who call themselves *Women in Midstream*, and the hundreds who have written us letters and answered our questionnaires. So let me start by thanking all these participants.

I found the *YWCA Ad Hoc Menopause Study Group* while their first major project, the writing and distribution of a questionnaire about menopause, was under way. My job as a part-time teacher had just fizzled out, so I was looking around for some worthwhile work to do. I was also beginning to experience unexplained hot-cheek flushes occasionally, so when I read about the YWCA group in a local newspaper, it sounded like the place for me.

I remembered the YWCA (Young Women's Christian Association) from my own school days at the University of Washington thirty years before as a group of dedicated and sober young women concerned with social issues. They had been housed with the Young Men's Christian Association in a building on a quiet corner of the campus.

My memories had not prepared me for the 1970s YWCA, however. I found a group of lively, young feminists, now separated from their male counterparts, working on the second floor of a building in the noisy middle of Seattle's University District, involved with such projects as a women's health clinic (Aradia), a rape relief counselling service, and a Third World women's resource center.

What was a menopause study group doing here? I learned that one or two of the middle-aged women on the YWCA's board of directors had asked one evening, "What are we doing for older women? We have some problems too, you know." With that, the menopause group was formed. It was "ad hoc" to begin with because nobody knew what would come of it. Though the group has been comprised mainly of women, ranging in age from forty-five to sixty, the younger women at the YWCA have always shown an interest in what we were doing, not only for themselves, they said, but because many had mothers who were suffering a variety of strange symptoms.

When I walked in that first day, I found three or four women trying to dig their way out from under stacks of mail. A story about the group and its questionnaire had been publicized by Isabella Taves in her syndicated newspaper column, "Women Alone," and requests for the questionnaires had inundated the small, volunteer staff.

"Thank goodness, her column appears only in modest-sized towns," one of the women said. "If she ran in New York, we'd be all through before we start." At that, besides Seattle, letters came from all over the country—from Binghamton, New York, to Denver, Colorado, to Hermosa Beach, California.

As a crash orientation course, someone handed me a stack of letters, saying, "Read these. They'll give you an idea of what we're up against."

The group had certainly hit a nerve. Many of the letters left me wondering and worrying—
about the bitterness:

> "This letter barely skims over the surface of my medical experiences equal to 'Terrors of Tess' . . . ten months of no treatment, maltreatment, and mistreatment."

about the loneliness:

> "I had a rough time going through menopause and very little help from any doctor—or anybody."

about the anxiety:

"I am not at the age of menopause, but I am in my late thirties, will be forty soon, and have heard so many tales."

Within a few weeks, that small volunteer staff mailed out over 1200 questionnaires. Eventually, over 700 replies came back. As we read them over, it became clear that many of the questions had been poorly phrased. They had been compiled by a committee of women interested in menopause but inexperienced with questionnaires.

Some questions asked for answers that were too subjective: "Is (or was) your menopause experience: easy, moderately easy, difficult, moderately difficult." Others were too general to be informative: a list of symptoms with directions to circle "any that have troubled you in the past or that currently trouble you."

Some questions that might have elicited valuable information had not been asked at all, for instance, specific details about the kinds of hormones women were taking and their dosages. Another we have been asked about would be a comparison between a woman's own experiences with menopause and her mother's. (We did ask these questions in a subsequent newsletter, but we received too few answers to be of value.) A copy of the complete questionnaire appears on page 146.

The Study group managed to collect enough money to have 250 of the questionnaires analyzed by computer. Though some of the information proved to be of general interest, we decided that most of the results were probably of slight scientific value because our sample had not been broad enough — the women who had requested questionnaires were a highly selective group with troublesome symptoms to begin with.

Some of the more general results were of significance, however, as we reported to the respondents in a newsletter.

GENERAL PROFILE

The majority of the respondents are married, live with their husbands and have children. The majority also work outside the home. All have experienced some menopausal symptoms. (What does this say about the oft-repeated assertion, "If only women would keep busy, they wouldn't be bothered by menopause"?)

Women are self-deprecating.

To the question, "Do you work outside the home?" many answered, "No, but I do volunteer work." Maybe the question was ambiguous—or maybe we need to straighten out in our heads just what "work" is.

Women tend to be martyrs about physical ailments.

Many rated their menopausal experiences as "easy" or "moderately easy," then checked off several distressing symptoms. We wonder what it takes to be "difficult"? Also, while 65% said they were "satisfied with their doctor's attitude," only 33% rated their doctor as "helpful." Another question, why don't we expect more from our doctors?

The questionnaire was just a beginning. We needed more information to answer responsibly the increasing numbers of questions we were hearing. It was also time for the ad hoc group to become permanent and to change its name. Since "menopause" suggested only a physical condition, we decided to change to a broader title, to indicate that we were concerned with all aspects of a woman's life during the middle years. One cannot separate physical from emotional and psychological states.

During one of those sessions when everyone tosses suggestions around, someone came up with "midstream," as an adaptation of "mid-life" and "mainstream." It sounded fresher than "mature women" or "changing years," so we became *Women in Midstream.*

Our first order of business was to gather all the information we could find by reviewing medical and popular publications, by interviewing doctors and health-care workers, and by talking with still more women.

Several letter-writers had warned us that published information was not easy to come by. One woman wrote, "I am fifty and going through menopause. After trips to the library I find that if I have a heart condition, ulcers, babies, dandruff, or hangnails, I am in good shape. But if I want some information on what's happening here and now, the well is dry." Another said, "About four years ago, I asked at the Minneapolis Public Library, surely one of the largest in the United States, about books on menopause—since I couldn't find any on the shelves. Imagine my surprise when the librarian went back to the stacks for the few she had! She just shrugged when I asked why. Are they classified as dirty books?"

When we started interviewing doctors, we were in for another surprise. They disagree sharply about the symptoms, the duration, and the treatment of menopause. And our reading left us even more confused. After learning to decipher the technical language of medical journals, we found contradictions and uncertainties there too.

Most popular books and magazines are even worse. They either make unrealistic promises: Estrogen will keep your skin forever as elastic as well-chewed bubble gum. Or they try to jolly women out of their anxieties: "There is nothing that can rival a rosy dawn and a flaming sunset as does that gift of the menopause, the hot flash." Or they provide helpful hints to live by: "Do something positive to overcome periods of depression. The old antidote of going out to buy a new hat is still great."

Why the lack of sensible information? To begin with, the whole study of the endocrine gland system, with its vital but complex hormone secretions, is quite recent. The female hormones, estrogen and progesterone, were not isolated and identified until 1929, and were only made available as medication when they were produced in crystalline form in the 1930s.

Another reason for the general lack of research about menopause was articulated recently by a physician who told us, "You must remember, women don't die from menopause. Medical researchers have been concentrating upon more serious physical ailments." Comments like this make some wonder whether there's not also a hard core of sexism in the neglect of the subject. Perhaps such a general accusation is unfair, but certainly many male doctors who have written about menopause have revealed an insensitivity toward older women which would raise the hackles of any thoughtful person.

Dr. Robert A. Wilson, an early advocate of hormone therapy, wrote in *Feminine Forever*, "A woman's body is the key to her fate. . . . Her physical, social, and psychological fulfillment all depend on one crucial test: her ability to attract a suitable male and to hold his interest over many years."

Dr. Howard W. Jones, Acting Director of the Department of Obstetrics and Gynecology, Johns Hopkins University, is quoted in an HEW pamphlet on *Menopause and Aging* as having characterized menopausal women as being "a caricature of their younger selves at their emotional worst."

And Dr. David Reuben of *Everything-You-Always-Wanted-to-Know-About-Sex* fame wrote, "As the estrogen is shut off, a woman comes as close as she can to being a man. . . . Not really a man, but no longer a functional woman, these individuals live in the world of intersex."

But women themselves must also share the blame for a lack of interest in menopause research. Too many want to avoid the whole subject. Several have reacted to the YWCA's study with disdain: "Ugh, save me from such depressing females," one said recently. "I suppose they all wear blue to your meetings—that's the menopause color, you know." Another returned one of our newsletters with a message scrawled across it, "Stuff this garbage!"

We decided the best way to answer put-downs like these would be to write a book ourselves—by women, about women. There was no trouble agreeing upon goals: "We would summarize and document current information, we would tell how other women feel about their experiences, and we would point to directions that women might take for themselves in the future.

I agreed to do the writing. The others would help with the research and interviews. We also decided to quote freely from the questionnaires and correspondence because so many women had expressed the hope that the sharing of their experiences might lead to answers which would make things easier for others. We have used fictitious names, however, to protect the privacy of our correspondents.

We decided on the title, *The Other Awkward Age*, not to put down middle-aged women (we've had enough of that already), but to emphasize the essential nature of the experience. It is a time, like the first awkward age of adolescence, when the body's hormone balance gets out of kilter. Fortunately, also like adolescence, menopause is a temporary condition. As the estrogen production of the ovaries diminishes and menstrual periods cease, a woman's body gradually adjusts to its new status. Many women go through the experience with little trouble, and most welcome the end of the general monthly nuisance. But a significant number of women do suffer considerable discomfort. By and large, it is these women we have heard from.

Let me add one warning about our book. Many vital questions about menopause remain to be answered. In putting this book together, we have had to learn to cope with exasperating differences of opinion on such important subjects as: What are menopausal symptoms? Should women take hormones? How long should hormone therapy be continued?

Of course, we do not advocate treatments. But we have gathered the most recent and most authoritative information we could find. All this is summarized here so that each reader may ask the appropriate questions about herself and may make sensible decisions about her own health.

Though our main purpose is to provide women with the information and reassurance they have so urgently requested, we address our book to others too: to the young women who have asked us what their futures hold; to the men who wonder about their wives' and mothers' experiences; and to the doctors who will be facing more women who will be asking more questions and demanding more answers.

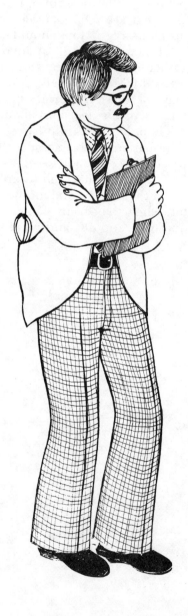

1
What Goes On Behind The Sheet?

Over and over again women have expressed unhappiness about their relations with doctors. This imaginary conversation between two friends, waiting in a busy clinic's reception room, reflects this irritation.

"When doctors say they *practice* medicine, they're not kidding, are they? I think they're a lot to blame for women's anxieties about menopause. They don't seem to know what to tell us."

"I don't care about facts so much. It's my doctor's general attitude that gets me. He acts so nonchalant about it all. Last time I was in the office, complaining about how tired I get, he said, 'Well, my dear, what do you expect—at your age?'"

"You should have said, 'Gee, I don't know, Doctor, I've never been this age before.'"

"I wouldn't dare. He doesn't have much of a sense of humor. In fact, he even gets irritated when I start asking questions."

"My God, isn't that what you're paying him for? I think women should know a whole lot more about their bodies than they do. Why, my fourteen-year-old daughter knows way more than I do even now."

"Well, I'm going to have to find it out from someone besides my doctor, then. He hardly has time to look at my body, let alone listen to me."

As letters and requests for information have come into the office, we have filed them according to subject. The fattest folder of all contains complaints about doctors. These range from mild dissatisfaction—"Even my own family doctor, who explains everything else asked of him at great length, doesn't seem to know what to say about menopause"—to grinding hostility—"I am fifty-four, active physically and mentally and resent being treated by my god-playing doctor as if I were a functional retardate or a dog in obedience school."

Some women recount specific complaints: "I have just had a hysterectomy and have been dumped surgically into menopause by a doctor who six weeks later *dismissed* me. Any information you could give me would probably help me sort out what happened."

Another young woman (thirty-two) who was experiencing menopausal symptoms after the removal of her uterus and ovaries wrote, "I have changed doctors because I got tired of hearing my first doctor tell me my only trouble was that I was bored. And I know I am not. He'd say, 'If you were fifty-five or sixty without small children, I'd tell you to stay in bed or knit all day when things seemed difficult. But since you can't do that, you'll have to grin and bear it."

Another woman told us that she felt brushed off. She had called her doctor because she was suffering from a severe stomach upset. He advised, "Get a bottle of Kaopectate. It's probably only the menopause."

A friend told us she had been dismissed from the hospital amid some confusion because her own doctor left on a vacation shortly after performing her hysterectomy, and the attending physician was unfamiliar with her case. A nurse had handed her a prescription for estrogen and told her to take the pills as directed. The only trouble was no one had given her any directions. She conscientiously took one every day for several months until a friend told her she probably should be taking a few days off every month. When she asked her doctor about it, he said, "Oh, yes, didn't I tell you? You should cycle them—three weeks on and one week off."

One correspondent wrote that she had experienced considerable anxiety because her doctor said, without further explanation, that if estrogen didn't help her, he would refer her to a psychiatrist. "This still worries me," she added.

Most of the criticisms we hear are not as specific as these. Many middle-aged women just feel that doctors aren't interested in explaining what they are doing. As one said, "I want information, not a pat on the hand."

Doctors must feel sometimes that they can't win. But they probably don't realize how intimidating and humiliating a physical examination can seem from the point of view of that sheet-shrouded patient on the table.

So we offer here the story of Genevra Gentless, another patient who had trouble bridging the gynecological gap. Women will understand. But how many doctors have thought of that "routine" office call from this perspective?

"Now, Mrs. Gentless, If you'll just take off everything but your shoes and put on the gown, Doctor will be right with you." The nurse gestured toward what looked to Genevra like a folded king-sized paper napkin on the examining table and backed out the door.

"Please. Just a minute, Miss Utter. How do you work this . . .?" Too late. Nurse Utter had firmly shut the door, leaving her patient in the sterile privacy of one of Dr. O. ver Bering's examining rooms, fumbling with a new-fangled disposable hospital gown.

As usual Genevra felt she had to hurry, lest the doctor arrive while she was half undressed. Maybe in her bra and panty hose. She always worried about embarrassing him by allowing herself to be seen in something other than the prescribed outfit. Not that she kidded herself that there was anything alluring any more about her fifty-one-year-old bulges and bumps. Even her most private body hair was getting gray.

But Dr. ver Bering always seemed a bit uncomfortable with the naked intimacy required for a general checkup. At first glance, he looked as mod as Dr. Welby's side-kick, with wrap-around glasses, sea-green surgeon's coat, and eggshell turtle-neck jersey. But his mustache, neatly cropped as Walter Pidgeon's, and his spine, stiff as General Westmoreland's, betrayed the doctor's essential conservatism. And though he addressed Genevra by her first name, when he could remember it, his eyes always focused on a point just halfway between her eyebrows and widow's peak, as if under the circumstances, he couldn't properly look at her, pupil to pupil.

Genevra laid her folded clothes on a straight-backed chair next to the table where medical instruments were arranged in careful order. She draped her navy cardigan over the pile to save the doctor the embarrassment of glimpsing a piece of her underwear. Still hurrying, and shivering now, even though the room must be eighty-seven degrees at least, she unfolded the gown. It reminded her of the ghost costumes she had made out of tissue paper for her two boys one Halloween. They hadn't worked out too well either. She never could decide whether the opening went in front or back, since it always seemed necessary for doctors to poke you from every angle. She finally decided to put it on like a coat and fold her arms. That way she could support her sagging midriff at the same time she held the thing together.

Genevra perched on the edge of the examining table, since her clothes covered the only chair. Miss Utter had said the doctor would be "right with her," but Genevra knew better. In the six years she had been seeing Dr. ver Bering for annual checkups, she figured she had waited altogether 374 minutes, counting reception and examining-room time. At that, she preferred going to an internist like him rather than an obstetrician-gynecologist because those women's specialists were forever having to rush off to the delivery room for unscheduled births.

She had forgotten to bring a magazine from the reception room and she had already memorized, during previous visits, the framed diplomas and licenses hanging on the walls. So this time Genevra counted the dots on the perforated ceiling tiles, trying to determine whether they were randomly patterned or whether each square had the same number. Her feet began to sweat and stick to the insides of her new Naturalizers. She studied her dangling, freshly-shaven legs, which looked for all the world like newly-varnished baseball bats, and started practicing to herself just how she would tell Dr. ver Bering about the difficulty that had developed during the last few months.

"Let's see, I'll lead up to it," she thought, "by saying I read in the *Good Housekeeping* medical column that sometimes women develop a certain dryness inside as they get older which makes sex uncomfortable, but usually hormones will help the condition. That way, maybe he won't ask me about my own experience at all."

At that moment, Genevra heard a quiet scratching outside, indicating that Dr. ver Bering was reviewing her records which Nurse Utter had stashed in the slot on the door. After a discreet knock and quiet cough, the doctor pushed in.

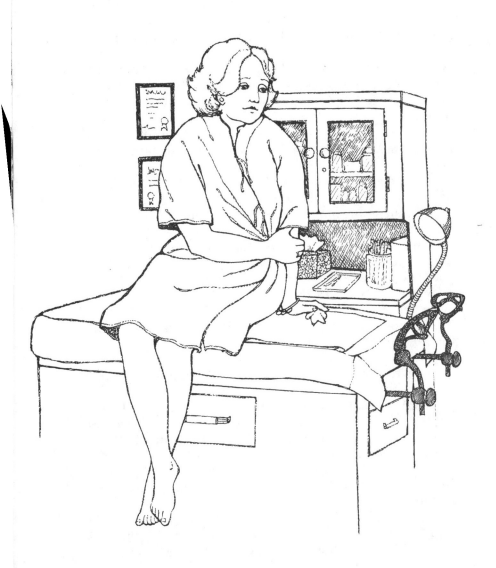

"Well, well," glancing quickly at her folder, "uh, Genevra, how are we feeling today?"

"Fine, Doctor, fine. Well, not really *fine*."

"Oh?" His eyes sought out that favorite spot on her forehead. "What seems to be the problem? Sit up straight and tell me all about it while I listen to your chest."

"Well, Doctor, I do seem to get tired awfully easily. By three in the afternoon . . ." Genevra let her voice trail off because Dr. ver Bering had plugged his ears with the stethoscope, and she didn't see how he could possibly hear her, even though he continued to nod encouragingly.

Unplugged now, he said, "You don't really feel fine, you say? Well, now, Gen-uh-my dear. Of course, as we get along in, uh, years, we can't always expect to be tiptop, can we? What exactly seems to bother you? Open your mouth, please." He flattened her tongue and peered down her throat with a flashlight.

"So far everything looks O.K. Are you ever troubled with dysmenorrhea, nocturia, or insomnia?"

Grasping at the only familiar word, Genevra stammered, "No, no, I usually sleep pretty well."

"What about hot flushes or night sweating? Have you noticed them yet?" A surreptitious glance at her card, "At your age . . ."

"My age," Genevra thought. "He makes me feel senile. What about his age?"

"No, not hot flushes," she said aloud. "But there is one thing I wanted to ask about."

"Yes? Lie down, please."

Genevra stretched out on her back and silently rehearsed her speech, while the doctor examined her breasts and prodded her abdomen. Somehow this didn't seem the time to tell him about it, not while he was feeling her all over. So Genevra silently counted the ceiling holes again.

Now Dr. ver Bering was draping her abdomen and thighs with a sheet. "Now, my dear, slide down the table, put your feet up in the stirrups, and relax," he directed, as he pulled on thin rubber gloves.

Genevra maneuvered herself around and placed her feet in the iron holders. Nurse Utter slipped through the door and stood at attention. The nurse's timing was always so exact, Genevra imagined that her heel touching the metal footrest set off warning lights at Miss Utter's desk, alerting her to stand by while the patient was in "the vulnerable position."

Miss Utter handed the doctor the instrument he used for peering up insides and whispered, "Mrs. Blackwell is ready now in room four, and Dr. Whitcomb wants you to call as soon as possible.

"Yes, yes, I'll be through here in a minute," the doctor answered under his breath. His head disappeared beneath the sheeted mound made by Genevra's knees. She winced as the cold metal touched her tender underside.

From below came Dr. ver Bering's voice. "One little thing troubling you, you say? This looks all right, Miss Utter. Swab for the Pap smear, please. What little thing is bothering you, Gen-uh?"

"Well, Doctor, sometimes when my husband and I . . . when we . . ." Genevra wished she could wait till Miss Utter had left. "When we're, you know, together. . . ." She swallowed to suppress a belch. When she got nervous like this, her stomach sent forth distress signals.

"Yes, go on." The doctor's disembodied voice rose from below. "When you and your husband?"

Genevra switched desperately to her planned strategy. "Well, Doctor, last week I read this article in *Good Housekeeping* about how women's membranes dry up some as they get older? And usually hormones . . ."

Dr. ver Bering's head rose like a blushing full moon between her sheeted knees. Was he flushed from crouching there below or was he irritated with her?

"Really, my dear, don't you ladies know that your physician doesn't have to hear about hormones from *Good Housekeeping*?" He snapped off his gloves and flung them into the waste basket.

"I know that, Doctor," Genevra apologized. "It's just that the article described so clearly the way I feel sometimes, well, during it."

Dr. ver Bering looked grave. "Sit up, please." His eyes slid away from her and concentrated on the ceiling. Was he counting the holes, too?

"You know, Genevra," (this time he got it right) "your husband . . . all men . . . have certain, uh, needs which must

15

be satisfied. Now, I'm going to prescribe these little pumpkin-seed pills—they're the hormones you read about. You take them as directed and let me know how you feel in four months. In the meantime . . ." Now he was backing out the door. "In the meantime, give your old man a break. Why not relax and enjoy it?"

To counter this catalog of patients' complaints, we interviewed a young woman gynecologist. Instead of trying to corner one of the offending doctors, we decided it would be more positive to talk with someone who might foreshadow a more enlightened future. Here is how she described her procedures.

Interviewer: We've told you about the complaints we hear from women about their doctors' attitudes. You were in medical school quite recently. Was this problem of communication with female patients ever discussed?
Doctor: Not really. What I do remember are the lewd jokes some of the male faculty told. Especially one who used nude pictures from *Playboy* magazine. Though, as I remember, he didn't discriminate. He showed nude men too.

Interviewer: You say you see mostly young women in your practice now?
Doctor: Yes, just a few older women. Because I'm working in family planning at the moment.

Interviewer: Do you ever feel that your patients are reticent or embarrassed about talking with you?
Doctor: No, usually it's just the opposite. They're so relieved to see another woman, they probably talk more than they would ordinarily. In fact, a lot of them state that specifically. A patient will say, "I've wanted to ask about this before but have been too embarrassed. It's really nice to be able to talk like this." Usually it has to do with their sexuality. Sometimes they have asked a doctor in the past and have felt so put down, they just shut up about it.

Interviewer: And you assume they were male doctors?
Doctor: I ask specifically. And usually it was a male. Occasionally it has been a woman doctor. But, of course, there aren't that many women doctors around.

Interviewer: What other complaints do you hear?

Doctor: Usually it has to do with lack of time—that doctors barely take time to explain what they're doing. And that they don't explain about medications they prescribe. Basically not explaining procedures.

Interviewer: In defense of these doctors, do you think they just don't have the time?

Doctor: That's true. Some get very busy and don't schedule enough time for each patient. On the other hand, some just don't want to do it. It does take a while to explain everything adequately.

Interviewer: Another complaint we hear is that doctors use such a complicated vocabulary, most lay people can't understand what they're saying anyway.

Doctor: Of course, doctors are so used to their terminology they don't stop to think a patient might not understand. And often the patient is too embarrassed to admit she doesn't understand.

Interviewer: That's one thing we can advise women to do. If you don't understand, be sure to ask. But I wonder whether sometimes doctors don't complicate their answers to cover up their own uncertainties.

Doctor: Yes, doctors are often uncomfortable admitting that they don't have absolute answers. It might weaken their authority.

Interviewer: And some women want to believe in that god-like image.

Doctor: They certainly feel more secure that way.

Interviewer: Now, would you describe just what you say to a woman when you see her for the first time, and what procedures you follow, especially in a pelvic exam?

Doctor: First, I will not allow a woman to be undressed and up in the stirrups as I walk in. She should be sitting down in a chair by my desk. If she's already undressed and in a gown, that's O.K., but I'd prefer that she be still in her street clothes. I go through her history. Find out whether she has any specific complaints. Then have her get undressed. Then I start the exam. First, I do a routine breast exam. Instruct her how to do that, if she hasn't learned how yet. Today most women have learned how. Unfortunately, I'm afraid most don't do it. Then I do the pelvic, explaining as I go along what I'm doing. And I always touch her leg before I start.

Interviewer: Why is that?
Doctor: So she'll get used to my touching her. And also it gives me an idea of how tense she is. If she's really anxious about it.

Interviewer: And if she seems anxious?
Doctor: I take more time. Explain constantly what I'm doing. Really talk through what I'm doing.

Interviewer: You explain about the instrument you use in the vagina?
Doctor: The speculum? Yes, I show it to her and tell her that I'm going to warm it before it touches her. I also tell her I'm not going to hurt her. Often the response is, "Doesn't it have to hurt?" Of course, it does hurt if she's tense, but it doesn't have to be painful. I offer her a mirror, if she would like to see her anatomy. Women who are nervous usually don't want that. That's fine. But those who are interested in looking become involved in what I'm doing and much more relaxed.

Interviewer: What about the sheets to cover her? Do you do that?
Doctor: I offer her a drape, if she's more comfortable with it. But I put it on in such a way that it doesn't obscure eye contact. If the patient can't see the person examining her, she just lies there and looks up at the ceiling. And that means nothing to her.

Interviewer: In fact, it's even more nerve-wracking.
Doctor: I've heard of one medical school where all the male students had to get on an examining table and put their feet in the stirrups.

Interviewer: What a good idea. Men just don't experience that indignity, do they?
Doctor: They have no idea what it feels like.

Interviewer: And often a woman first sees the doctor from that embarrassing position.
Doctor: No wonder she feels anxious and vulnerable.

Interviewer: And foolish.
Doctor: Another thing. I always give the patient some tissues after the exam. You would be surprised how often that's forgotten. She's got lubricating jelly all over her. That doesn't feel too great, if she can't wipe herself off. Then I also help her off the table. It is easy to slip.

Interviewer: Is it a law that a nurse must always be in attendance during a pelvic exam? Lots of women believe it is.
Doctor: It's usually a hospital regulation or just the doctor's policy for his own protection. So a patient can't claim he assaulted her, I suppose. Of course, it's not done if it's a woman doctor examining a man.

Interviewer: Apparently men don't feel vulnerable?
Doctor: Or they wouldn't object? I don't know why. Anyway, to sum up, my principal aim is to treat each patient with consideration and make her feel at ease, so she will tell me exactly what is on her mind—what might be troubling her.

Interviewer: Thanks so much, Doctor. I think you've given us an ideal against which to measure others' procedures.

Having outlined some of the general roadblocks women encounter in trying to communicate with their doctors, we will next describe just what does go on in the female body during menopause, what changes occur that may trigger some of those peculiar symptoms.

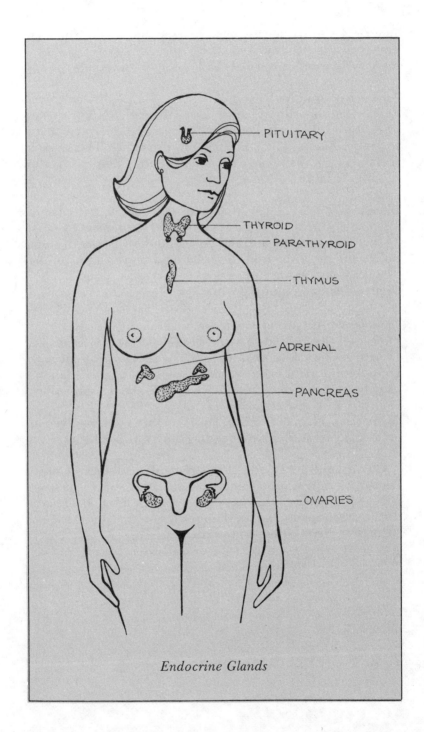

Endocrine Glands

2

What Does Menopause Mean?

Wanda pulled off her jacket and draped it over the back of her chair, saying, "Phew. It is too warm in here, isn't it, Bette?"

"It sure feels that way to me. This room could use a new ventilation system, if you ask me."

The two friends were visiting during a coffee break in the employee lounge.

"That's a relief," Wanda said. "I've gotten to the place where I don't even mention it any more if I get too warm in the office. The girls always laugh about Wanda's 'grand climacteric.' "

"I wonder why people so often make fun of menopausal symptoms? They wouldn't laugh if you said you had a headache or even menstrual cramps."

"It does seem mean, come to think of it. Maybe it's just because they're embarrassed. Don't know what else to say."

"Or maybe they take their cues from women themselves. Lots of us who are sensitive about it make a joke to cover our embarrassment. I know I do," Bette admitted.

"It's all part of our dread of getting old, I guess. You hate to admit it's finally happening to you. I remember when I was a kid, I used to hear my mother's friends talking. You know, when I wasn't supposed to be listening? I'd hear all that stuff about hot flashes and night sweats and think, 'Phooey! I'm not going to get old and sound like that.' So it really shook me up when I started feeling flushed and sweaty. And at such inconvenient times. The first real hot flush I had was when I was being interviewed for this job. I was so embarrassed. But looking back now, I bet Mr. Willis didn't even notice. At least he hired me anyway."

"He probably thought, 'Now here's a mature woman I can depend on. She won't quit after six months to have a baby.' But

seriously, I think stress has a lot to do with causing hot flushes. At least it makes them worse."

"I first noticed that I'd get too warm at night in bed. Sometimes I'd sleep with my feet dangling over the edge of the bed."

"What bugs me is how irritable I get. I just can't seem to control my temper sometimes. The other night I got one of those advertising phone calls at dinnertime, offering me a color portrait, absolutely free. I yelled, 'Well, you know what you can do with your picture. I'm cooking.' I bet that sweet young thing on the phone didn't know ladies talked like that."

"And the spells of anxiety you go through. And over the weirdest things. The last time we took a ferry ride, I was so sure that boat would sink that I didn't dare get out of the car. Luckily the ride lasted only twenty minutes. My sister thinks I'm a baby. She says she never noticed anything when she went through menopause. She just stopped menstruating."

"All that proves is everybody's different. I've got to get back to work, but first I want to tell you about one good symptom. My neighbor says she's been having really erotic dreams since she started having hot flushes."

"Say, Bette, maybe we could work on that one."

Not all young women are as flippant abut menopause as Wanda's coworkers. Recently we asked a community college class, where we had gone to present our program, what they thought happens during menopause. Here are some of their responses:

"I'm eighteen and never really thought about it, a scary experience maybe?" "I'm not worried about menopause. I'm going to get through it using hormones." "Menopause will be a time when my body goes through a chemical change. I will no longer have a period (thank heavens) and I will not be able to have children (thanks again)." "My mother is having a rough time now with it. I only hope I don't suffer the way she is." "I expect an extended feeling similar to what happens to me the few days before my period—anxiety, supersensitivity, crying for no reason. But I also will know that it's a physical-chemical change and not in my head. I'm not afraid of it."

These young women's comments typify the conflicting opinions we have run into throughout our research. About the only thing on which there is general agreement is the word itself: *menopause — permanent cessation of the menses; termination of the menstrual life.*

Then the differences of opinion begin to show up. You will find that many dictionaries and even some medical people use the term *climacteric* as a synonym for *menopause,* but *Stedman's Medical Dictionary* makes a distinction between the words: *climacteric — a period of life occurring in women preceding termination of the reproductive period and characterized by endocrine* [glandular] *somatic* [bodily], *and psychic changes, and ultimately menopause.* We mention this difference in terminology to explain the kind of statement we heard recently from a doctor who said that the climacteric may last for three to four years, while the menopause occurs in just a few months. In our book, however, we will use the single word *menopause* to describe the whole period.

Though menopause is a natural process, an inevitable aspect of aging, which usually occurs between the ages of forty-eight and fifty-two, each woman experiences it in an individual way. Such variations should not be surprising when one considers how differently women's bodies respond to other physical functions — like puberty, menstruation, pregnancies, and births.

Menopause usually develops gradually. A woman will notice an increasing irregularity in her monthly cycle. She may occasionally skip periods or the menstrual flow may become erratic — either lighter or heavier than usual. Finally she will stop menstruating altogether. After one year without menstrual periods, a woman may assume the menopausal process is complete.

What brings on menopause in the first place?

In simplest terms, menopause occurs because the ovaries no longer produce the hormones, *estrogen* and *progesterone,* in quantities sufficient to stimulate and to regulate the menstrual cycle.

When a woman is born, her ovaries contain about one-half million eggs. During her child-bearing years several of these eggs develop each month in sacs called *follicles,* but normally only one egg (an ovum) matures and is released to travel through a Fallopian tube to the uterus. The other partially developed egg sacs wither away. While the egg sacs develop, they produce increasing amounts of the hormone, estrogen, which begins to prepare the uterus for the eventual arrival of the ovum. After the ovum is released, its follicle produces progesterone, a second hormone which works with estrogen to enrich the uterine lining (the endometrium) for the implantation of a fertilized ovum. If the ovum is not fertilized, the uterine lining and the ovum are sloughed off in a menstrual period and the progesterone supply is cut down until the next cycle.

The exact reason for the gradual slow-down and eventual cessation in the function of the ovaries has not been definitely determined, but most researchers believe it is associated with the depletion of the supply of follicles, which, in turn, suppresses the supply of estrogen. As the estrogen diminishes, progesterone is no longer produced in quantities sufficient to enrich the uterine lining, so menstrual periods cease.

What are the symptoms of menopause?

To begin with, half of the women who go through menopause have few, if any, troublesome symptoms. Probably in these cases their estrogen supply drops so gradually that the body has time to adjust to the new hormonal levels with little disruption. There is some evidence that the ovaries may continue producing a diminishing supply of estrogen for many years after menstrual periods cease. Also the adrenal glands may supply small amounts of estrogen indefinitely.

Even those women with more severe problems will certainly not experience all the symptoms which have been associated with menopause. But we want to emphasize that these problems are real. Most of them have identifiable physical causes. And those which do develop from emotional or psychological stress should not be laughed away as imaginary complaints of aging, idle females whose health would improve if they would only find something to keep them busy. As one of our correspondents wrote, "I do 'keep busy,' involved in several organizations, as well as carrying twelve credits at college, plus three children. However, the symptoms are nonetheless real and severe. I begin to feel I am at the whim and will of my hormones, to say nothing of an unsympathetic medical profession."

This woman was correct in recognizing the power of her hormones—those potent chemical substances which are carried through the blood stream. A diminished supply of estrogen might well have widespread effects upon the body.

This is because the ovaries' production of estrogen is stimulated and regulated through a complex interaction between the ovaries and the pituitary gland, which is situated at the base of the brain and has been called the master gland of the whole endocrine system. When the ovaries slow down their production of estrogen, the pituitary gland becomes unusually active in secreting large amounts of one of its hormones (FSH —follicle stimulating hormone) which stimulates the ovaries. The pituitary, in turn, is regulated by the hypothalamus, that section of the brain just above the pituitary, which controls such functions as sleep, heat regulation, energy levels, the involuntary nervous system, and the emotions. When this delicately balanced system is thrown out of kilter by the ovaries' slowdown, a woman's whole body might well reflect the results.

With hot flushes (or flashes), for example. We prefer the term *flush* because it describes the sensation of overall blushing so well. Although their exact cause is not completely understood, many doctors believe these periods of warm flushing, sometimes followed by cold sweats (one of our correspondents described her chills as "ice-cube" flashes), are a reflection of this temporary disruption in the complex interaction between the hypothalamus, the pituitary, and the ovaries. One medical report on the subject states, "This symptom may be triggered by emotional stress, exercise, eating, or any factor that affects the mechanism of heat loss, such as lying in bed under a blanket or sitting in a warm room."

Another reason for the widespread impact of the diminishing estrogen supply upon the body involves the numerous functions of the hormone itself. Besides regulating the reproductive system, estrogen also affects skin tone. After menopause a woman will probably notice that her skin has become drier and less elastic. What happens on the outside of the body, happens on the inside too, with membranes drying and thinning out. The reproductive tract is especially affected. The ovaries and the uterus gradually shrink and the vagina becomes narrower, somewhat more rigid, and less able to secrete lubricating fluids. Breast tissue may become softer.

Both female and male sex hormones are produced naturally in women as well as men, with the appropriate one dominating in each sex. While in a woman the male hor-

25

mones (androgens) are subordinated to the female hormones, the balance between them may shift slightly during menopause. This is probably the reason some women may notice an increase in body hair, especially on the face.

The medical profession generally agrees that three conditions—the cessation of menses, hot flushes, and the drying of skin and membranes—are caused by the lowered estrogen levels of menopause. But here consensus ends. Many doctors identify only these three symptoms as menopausal, while others believe many more middle-age problems are associated with the hormonal imbalance women experience at this time. For example, Dr. Helen Z. Jern, an endocrinologist who specializes in the treatment of menopausal patients, believes that estrogen has wide-ranging effects. She states in *Hormone Therapy of the Menopause and Aging*, "Estrogen also plays a vital role in body metabolic processes, and especially in the metabolism of protein and fat. Consequently, an adequate amount of estrogen in the body of a woman is necessary for maintaining the normal function of her every cell." She lists twenty-four different symptoms as menopausal; among them, nervousness, depression, insomnia, dizziness, headaches, exhaustion, and inability to cope with life, confusion, and lack of memory and concentration.

Two problems of aging—hardening of the arteries (arteriosclerosis) and thinning of the bones (osteoporosis)—are currently under special study because opinions about their causes seem to be changing. At one time researchers generally agreed that both conditions were directly related to lower levels of estrogen in older women. But now many believe the causes are more complex—that inadequate diet and diminished physical activity might be just as important to their development as lower estrogen supplies.

We cannot mediate medical disagreements, but we have learned through direct correspondence with several hundred women that many of them have experienced unfamiliar and irritating symptoms. For example, one woman wrote, "I had always been an extremely healthy, optimistic person with no fears of menopause. I was completely unprepared for the drastic series of conditions that came upon me."

Of the more than 700 who responded to the YWCA's questionnaire, 26.4% were troubled by insomnia, 26% with tension headaches, 23.2% with heart palpitations, and 18.8% with frequent urination.

26

In addition to these physical disturbances, even more women experienced emotional upsets: irritability, 37.6%; nervousness, 34.4%; depresssion, 33.6%; crying spells, 38%; and apprehension, 28%. Some wrote about "feeling pressure from trivial things," or "being very touchy, restless, and hard to get along with," or "experiencing a general feeling of hopelessness."

Of course, physical and emotional disturbances feed upon each other. A woman who is awakened frequently with hot flushes and profuse sweating will certainly suffer from insomnia and, no doubt, feel pretty irritable during the day. Conversely, medical researchers have found that stressful situations will make hot flushes more severe.

The most reassuring word we can offer is that many of these problems will gradually subside as the body adjusts to its new hormonal balance. And other, more persistent, symptoms can probably be treated by one of the several methods described in subsequent chapters.

What is involved in a pelvic examination?

Whether or not a woman is experiencing troublesome symptoms, she would be wise to have a pelvic examination at least once a year. To find out just why all that pushing and probing during such examinations is necessary, we asked our medical consultant to explain exactly what does go on. She also described two other important diagnostic techniques: the Pap smear and the D and C.

Interviewer: Doctor, will you tell us just what is involved in a routine pelvic exam?
Doctor: First, you start with the external inspection, examining the genitalia — the clitoris, the urethra, the labia majora, the labia minora — looking for any obvious abnormalities, like lesions or growths. Then check the Bartholin glands, which are located near the vaginal opening, and the periurethral glands to see if there might be a cyst or inflammation. Check for any abnormal discharge which the woman may not be aware of. You may also check for muscular support by asking the patient to bear down. This is to make sure the muscles and ligaments around the vagina are strong and elastic. Lack of good pelvic support may result in the uterus or bladder sagging or prolapsing into the vagina. If you find that the support is weak, you can give the patient some exer-

cises to strengthen those muscles to alleviate some problems later. This inspection of the external genitalia is very important. Most women don't look at themselves to see that everything looks normal. So I think a doctor should do this part very carefully.

Interviewer: Then you examine the patient inside?
Doctor: Yes, next comes the examination with the speculum. You put it into the vagina in order to visualize the walls of the vagina and the cervix and to collect specimens for lab tests. That is when you would take the Pap smear and gonorrhea culture. A lot of women assume that the Pap smear will also show any venereal disease, but that requires an entirely different test. Wet mounts for vaginitis are also done at this time, if it is necessary. Then you can take the speculum out and do the bimanual examination.

Interviewer: What does that mean?
Doctor: Simply, it means using two hands. It is done by putting two fingers of one hand into the vagina and placing the other hand on the outside of the abdomen and gently pushing the uterus down toward the inside examining fingers. The purpose is to outline the uterus and the ovaries to make sure they feel normal. You are concerned with the shape, position, size, and consistency of the uterus. The size can vary, of course, but if it seems abnormally large, you can assume that something is going on that should be checked further. You're also concerned with the consistency of the organ. If it feels boggy or soft, again you will suspect that something abnormal might be going on. You also look for tenderness. If there is any infection, the patient will feel tenderness from all the movement and palpation. Then you use your examining fingers to go over to each side of the pelvis and feel the ovaries. This is not always possible, but if the patient is relaxed and not too overweight, you can usually palpate them. The ovaries are almond-shaped and about the same size. Often the patient can communicate to you that you are feeling her ovaries because she will experience a characteristic kind of twinge. What you are checking for is to make sure there is no cyst or mass on the ovaries or around the Fallopian tubes. You cannot feel the tubes unless disease is present. So you're just generally checking the whole pelvic area to make sure there are no abnormalities that can be felt.

Interviewer: Does that complete the procedure then?
Doctor: Not quite. The other part of the pelvic exam, which is very important, is the rectal exam. And it is too often neglected, I'm afraid. This is done by inserting one finger in the rectum and one finger in the vagina simultaneously, examining the anal area and rectum, and again palpating the uterus and ovaries. The rectal exam enables you to feel behind the uterus, again to check for any abnormal growths there or on the rectum.

Interviewer: How long does the whole pelvic exam take?
Doctor: Even though it sounds complicated, it usually takes only four or five minutes to complete.

Interviewer: Do you think the exam should be done routinely once a year?
Doctor: Yes, once a year, assuming no medical problems occur during that time.

Interviewer: What about older women? Women past menopause?
Doctor: That depends. Some physicians advise yearly exams for these women as well. Others advise exams every six months.

Interviewer: Now will you explain how a Pap smear is done?
Doctor: You probably know that it is named for the man who developed the technique, Dr. Papanicolaou. The Pap smear has two parts. The first part is the cervical scrape. Here you are trying to obtain endocervical cells, which are up inside the cervical canal. Usually you use a wooden or plastic spatula. It goes inside the cervical opening, and scrapes the outer surface of the cervix as well. You turn it around 360 degrees, then spread that specimen on a slide and permanently fix it. What you are mainly looking for are changes in the endocervical cells. The most likely place for cancer of the cervix to develop is at the spot where the two different cell layers meet, up in the endocervical canal where cells from the outer cervix meet with the cells from the cervical canal.

Interviewer: Then what is the second part of the Pap smear?
Doctor: The second area that is sometimes sampled by the Pap smear is the vagina. This can sometimes pick up ab-

normal cells from the uterine lining which may have fallen into the vagina.

Interviewer: Now would you explain about a D and C? What it involves and what the indications are for having one?
Doctor: The *D* stands for *dilatation* which involves dilating or widening the cervical canal. And the *C, for curretage* which involves the scraping of the lining of the uterus. As to indications, it can be used for abortion procedures, to help diagnose why abnormal bleeding is occurring, or to remove and diagnose polyps or abnormal growths inside the uterus or endocervical canal. The tissue which has been removed is sent to a pathologist who will analyze the tissue to see whether any abnormalities exist.

Interviewer: Is a D and C performed in a hospital?
Doctor: It can be done in two different ways. The first is in an operating room with the patient under a general anesthetic. This is probably the most common way because the patient feels no discomfort. But even with a general anesthetic, more and more hospitals now have ambulatory surgical units, where the patient checks in and goes home on the same day. This saves the expense of staying overnight.

Interviewer: Then what is the second method?
Doctor: Many doctors, who are trying to lower the cost for the patient, are doing the D and C in their offices or in an out-patient facility, where they don't have to put the patient to sleep. They may give her a tranquilizer and then inject a local anesthetic around the cervix. This is usually left up to the discretion of the physician. If the physician thinks there might be a lot of tissue to be removed, a general anesthetic may be preferable. If it is necessary to take only a small sample of tissue, a local anesthetic may be sufficient. But both are essentially the same.

Interviewer: Then just how is the scraping done?
Doctor: First a clamp called a tenaculum is applied to the cervix, to hold and stabilize the cervix and uterus. Next a set of graduated dilators is used, ranging in diameter from 1/16 inch to 1/4 inch — making the opening large enough to insert the curette. There are two kinds of curettes. A sharp curette is

a spoon-shaped metal instrument with a sharp edge which is used to scrape the lining of the uterus to remove tissue. A suction curette is a flexible hollow plastic tube with an opening at the tip. The tube is attached to a vacuum and some of the tissue that lines the uterus is aspirated through the hollow tube. Either of these techniques can be used for the curettage.

Interviewer: If a woman has been having problems with heavy and irregular bleeding, will the D and C itself correct the problem?
Doctor: Sometimes it corrects it, but often only temporarily. If an abnormal build-up of the uterine lining occurs, which sloughs off with a heavy period, it may start building up again after the D and C.

Interviewer: Are D and Cs repeated then?
Doctor: They can be. But the concern is that symptoms of abnormal bleeding may be caused by cancer of the endometrium, especially among women who are post menopausal. So it is very important to make a proper diagnosis. That's why physicians are very particular about doing a D and C if there is abnormal bleeding—either with spotting between periods or with heavy menstrual flow.

Interviewer: So it is important for women, especially during or after menopause, to check out any unusual bleeding which may occur.
Doctor: Absolutely. Without exception. I can't emphasize that point strongly enough.

● For those women who do not do a monthly breast self-examination because they have forgotton how, here are the instructions of the American Cancer Society:

1. *In the Shower:*
   Examine your breasts during bath or shower; hands glide easier over wet skin. Fingers flat, move gently over every part of each breast. Use right hand to examine left breast, left hand for right breast. Check for any lump, hard knot, or thickening.

2. *Before a Mirror:*
   Inspect your breasts with arms at your sides. Next, raise your arms high overhead. Look for any changes in contour of each breast, a swelling, dimpling of skin, or changes in the nipple.

   Then, rest palms on hips and press down firmly to flex your chest muscles. Left and right breast will not exactly match—few women's breasts do.

   Regular inspection shows what is normal for you and will give you confidence in your examination.

3. *Lying Down:*
   To examine your right breast, put a pillow or folded towel under your right shoulder. Place right hand behind your head—this distributes breast tissue more evenly on the chest. With left hand, fingers flat, press gently in small circular motions around an imaginary clock face. Begin at outermost top of your right for 12 o'clock, then move to 1 o'clock, and so on around the circle back to 12. A ridge of firm tissue in the lower curve of each breast is normal. Then move in an inch, toward the nipple, keep circling to examine *every part of your breast*, including nipple. This requires at least three more circles. Now slowly repeat procedure on your left breast with a pillow under your left shoulder and left hand behind head. Notice how your breast structure feels.

   Finally, squeeze the nipple of each breast gently between thumb and index finger. Any discharge, clear or bloody, should be reported to your doctor immediately.

You should do the exam about a week after each menstrual period. Or if you no longer have periods, do it at a regular time, like the first of every month. Remember, ninety percent of breast changes are found by women themselves. Most of them are not malignant. But the earlier cancer is detected, the greater the chance of cure.

In 1976 some questions developed about the advisability of doing periodic breast X-rays (mammograms) on all women, like those being done in twenty-seven cancer detection centers across the country, because of the danger of exposure to excess amounts of radiation over the years. In August 1976 the National Cancer Institute and the American Cancer Society issued a joint statement, recommending that women under fifty years of age should avoid such routine mammograms. Only those women with suspicious breast conditions or those considered to be in a high-risk category — with a previous history of breast cancer themselves or with a strong family history of the disease — should be given mammograms, the organizations stated. They did recommend, however, that women over fifty, whose risk is higher because the incidence of the disease increases with age, should continue having periodic mammograms.

But many doctors question whether all women over fifty need to have regular mammograms; they would continue to reserve the X-ray for suspicious cases. This is something each woman should decide in consultation with her own doctor.

But whatever her age or whatever other techniques are used, every woman should examine her own breasts every month.

We decided we should not try to discuss in this book the different types of breast surgery being performed today. It is such a controversial and rapidly changing situation that we could not report it fully enough to present an authoritative picture. A cancer specialist we interviewed emphasized that the breast contains some of the most complex tissues in the body. It is, therefore, impossible to generalize about breast disease or treatment, he said. Diagnoses and decisions about procedures must be made on individual cases, based on that individual's past history and present condition.

However, some informative books for the lay person have been published on the subject in recent years. We have included several in the Suggested Readings List.

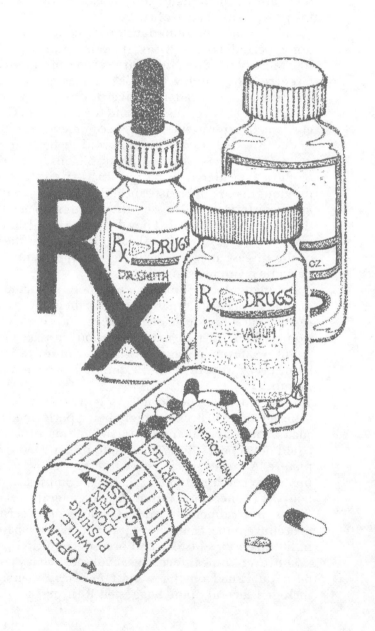

3

What About Hormone Therapy?

*I read in the paper that some doctors
think these hormone pills aren't safe
for treating menopause. As long as there's
any question, I've decided not to take
them at all. Why not just let nature
take its course—*
From a letter to *Women in Midstream*

For more than thirty years the most popular treatment for
the relief of menopausal symptoms has been *estrogen replacement therapy* (ERT). Under this regimen a woman's
naturally diminishing supply of the female hormone is
replenished through shots or pills of estrogen. The hormone
may be obtained from a number of sources. Some are manufactured chemically and are called synthetic. Others are
extracted from animal sources (usually from the urine of
pregnant mares) and are called natural conjugated estrogens.

There is little dispute that such hormones relieve the two
main menopausal symptoms—hot flushes and drying vaginal membranes. And some women believe they help in other
ways, like combatting insomnia and nervous tension.

What is the evidence against hormone therapy?
In the winter of 1975 alarm bells started jangling for mil-
lions of middle-aged women who had been confidently taking
estrogen, some for several years. That December newspapers
and magazines publicized two articles from *The New England*

Journal of Medicine which reported unsettling news about this therapy.

The first reported that the incidence of cancer of the lining of the uterus (the endometrium) had increased among women taking estrogen for menopausal symptoms. The study was based upon the records of some six hundred patients from three Seattle hospitals over a twelve-year period (1960-72). In fact, the indications were that the risk had increased as much as eight times.[1]

The second article reported that a similar increase had been reflected among women using natural conjugated estrogens (Premarin). It cited records of over three hundred patients from a Los Angeles medical center over a four-year period (1970-74).[2]

This disturbing news was slightly moderated by the knowledge, as outlined by Dr. Kenneth J. Ryan in an editorial in the same journal, that cancer of the uterus is still a relatively rare form of the disease. Also, as Dr. Noel S. Weiss stated in a second editorial, many complicating factors still remain to be analyzed. Among them, whether the amount of estrogen taken and the duration of treatment will influence the possible risks of cancer.

Since Dr. Donald C. Smith, one of the authors of the first report, practices in Seattle at the Mason Clinic, we immediately arranged to interview him. He told us that his phone had been ringing off the wall since the news stories about his article had appeared in local papers. All his colleagues in the clinic had been kept busy reassuring their patients too. They agreed that there was no immediate cause for alarm.

Dr. Smith emphasized that a retrospective, statistical study like the one he participated in does not establish causation. There is no way to tell whether those patients in the study would have developed endometrial cancer anyway. All it indicates is there is an increased relative risk of developing it among women who take estrogen. Also the Seattle women used several different kinds of estrogens, so all types seemed to be implicated. The California study dealt with Premarin, he said, probably because that was the kind used at the Kaiser Hospital.

As far as his own practice is concerned, Dr. Smith told us that he has not stopped prescribing estrogen therapy for

---

1   Donald C. Smith, M.D.
2   Harry K. Ziel, M.D.

those patients who require it. After all, any medication involves risks as well as benefits, he reminded us. However, not all women need additional estrogen. And for those who do take it, he keeps the dosage as low as possible (0.3 mg to 0.625 mg of Premarin or its equivalent in other pills) and encourages his patients to cut down on that quantity after a few months, with the goal of stopping altogether when they can do that comfortably.

Dr. Smith concluded the interview with the reassurance that there is now a great impetus to investigate the whole subject more thoroughly, and that he believes much will be learned in the next few years.

Shortly after this interview, we discovered that Dr. Noel S. Weiss, who wrote one of the editorials in *The New England Journal*, commenting on these findings, is also in Seattle, as a faculty member of the University of Washington Medical School. So next we made an appointment to talk with him. He speaks from the point of view of an epidemiologist, a researcher involved with statistical studies of larger populations than a practicing physician would see. It was because of this perspective that he was asked to comment upon the two articles, he explained.

First, he said it seemed logical that estrogen had the potential of causing cancer because of the nature of the hormone itself. It stimulates the growth of cells, particularly those of the uterine lining. Also within the last ten to fifteen years estrogens have been used more widely than before in treating menopausal patients. The sales of estrogens have increased two to three times in the past ten years. And an increase in the rate of the incidence of uterine cancer has paralleled this rise in estrogen use. Such statistics, added to the results of Dr. Smith's and Dr. Ziel's studies, seem very persuasive, he said.

However, Dr. Weiss also believes that, in balance, estrogen may do more good than harm in relieving problems which may develop during the menopausal years. That is one subject that must be studied more thoroughly, he added — exactly what the benefits of estrogen therapy may be. Another point to be considered is that endometrial cancer generally has a high rate of cure. Furthermore, the type which seems to develop under estrogen stimulation is possibly not as malignant as other uterine cancers.

Like Dr. Smith, Noel Weiss also emphasized that much more must be learned about the whole subject.He is presently involved in conducting a study in the Seattle area. Its aim is to identify all women in King County who develop uterine cancer during an eighteen-month period and to compare them with a representative sample of healthy women. They will all be interviewed in detail about their use of estrogens—the dosage, type of medication, and duration of therapy. A pathologist is checking the cancer specimens to identify the incidence of different types.

Dr. Weiss assured us that studies like these, and the numerous similar ones which will be conducted throughout the country, should produce the additional data required to develop more beneficial treatment programs within the next few years.

Six months later two more articles on the subject appeared in the same medical journal (June 1976). One by Dr. Weiss presented further statistical evidence regarding uterine cancer's increase. The second, by Dr. Thomas M. Mack of the University of Southern California, based upon a study of women in a California retirement community, confirmed the earlier findings of a probable relationship between estrogen therapy and uterine cancer. Dr. Mack added, however, that the risk seemed less when the hormone was taken in monthly cycles with intervals of four or more days between without the medication.

Why is there so much disagreement?

Calm, objective assessments like those provided in the interviews with Drs. Smith and Weiss can be at once reassuring and frustrating. The statistics sound scientific enough, but what should each individual woman do? Why can't doctors give better answers? Why doesn't the medical profession know more about hormones and menopause anyway?

To begin with, one must remember the intricate functions of the endocrine system (as described in Chapter Two). The glands operate in a very delicate balancing act, with the functions of one gland influencing another. More needs to be known, for example, about the effects on a menopausal woman's body of the higher levels of the pituitary gland's hormonal output as it tries to stimulate the failing ovaries to produce more estrogen.

A further complication involves the nature of estrogen itself. Though it is often referred to as a single hormone, there are actually several different kinds of estrogens. The three types identified so far have been named estrone, estradiol and estriol. It is now believed that each of these estrogens might have a specialized function which has not yet been exactly determined.

During menopause the balance among these three types of estrogen probably changes. As the ovaries shut down their supply of estrogens, the adrenal glands become the main source of the hormone, and they produce mainly estrone. A recent study suggests that this increased supply of estrone during the menopausal years may be implicated in a woman's increased susceptibility to uterine cancer as she grows older.

Another change in a menopausal woman's hormonal balance involves the decrease in the second main group of ovarian hormones, the progestins. Like the estrogens, there are probably several types of progestins, but the main one is progesterone. Not much is known about its functions other than its role in inducing menstrual periods. It is often referred to as having an anti-estrogenic effect because it is involved in triggering the shedding of the uterine lining which has been enriched by the action of estrogen. Apparently, after menopause, the body produces little or no progesterone, so the estrogen which is supplied, whether naturally or as medication, is no longer counteracted or opposed by progesterone. This is another important difference in an older woman's hormonal environment.

Add to this complex picture the individual differences which exist among women, and one begins to understand why doctors sometimes seem a bit vague in their answers to specific questions. An individual's exact estrogen level is difficult to determine. The vaginal smear, which is usually taken at the time of the Pap test, measures only extremes of estrogen levels. Blood and urine tests, which may also be used for measurement, are complicated and expensive. And all labs are not equipped to do them. One researcher explained to us that the body naturally produces only infinitesimal amounts of estrogen. Even the smallest doses given for therapy represent much higher levels than occur naturally. "It is like killing a fly with a sledge hammer," he said. Furthermore, no estrogen, whether from an animal source or

synthetically produced, which may be administered to re-
place the body's diminishing natural supply, exactly matches,
in the same proportions, all the elements in the body's own
hormones.

As noted in Chapter Two, there is also considerable dis-
agreement as to just how estrogen functions. Is it involved in
all aspects of metabolism in the body, as Dr. Helen Jern believes? Or is its function simply the regulation of the reproductive system? These questions are crucial because those
doctors who believe that estrogens have wide-ranging effects
upon the body will be more likely to advise a patient that the
benefits of hormone therapy outweigh the risks than those
who believe an estrogen deficiency causes nothing more
than transitory discomforts. This fundamental assumption
will also influence a doctor's attitude as to how long hormone
therapy should be continued. One who believes that the
female hormones have a continuing influence throughout
the body would logically advise a woman to continue replacement therapy indefinitely.

How do doctors decide what to prescribe?

In order to better understand the wide differences of
opinion about hormone therapy within the medical profession and to explain the reasons for these differences, we
interviewed several doctors about their own beliefs and
treatment programs. We chose the types of specialists whom
we thought women would be most likely to consult: several
gynecologists and family medicine practitioners, an internist, and an endocrinologist. We talked with both female and
male doctors—some new to the practice of medicine, others
with years of experience. They were all cooperative and
encouraging about our project.

Of course, they were all aware of the recent findings asso-
ciating estrogen therapy with an increase in uterine cancer
and planned to tell their patients about them. But their reactions to the reports ranged from special concern to skepti-
cism. One gynecologist told us that she questioned the data
presented so far. Pathologists are identifying cellular altera-
tions in the endometrium as "cancer" much earlier in the
continuum of change than they used to. However, this early
diagnosis makes for very high cure rates. Another gynecologist reminded us that uterine cancer existed long before

estrogen therapy began, so we must not be too quick to accept a cause and effect relationship in the recent studies.

Each interview lasted from twenty to forty minutes. And each emphasized different aspects of the subject, depending upon the specialty involved. But we made sure to ask three basic questions:

1. How do you determine a patient's need for estrogen therapy and the dosage required?
2. What therapy program would you prescribe?
3. How long should a patient take hormones?

We quote here the answers from seven of the doctors—those which represent the widest range of opinion.

How do you determine the need for hormones, and the dosage?	*What treatment program do you recommend?*	*How long should therapy be continued?*

[1] DR. A (Female) Family Medicine, 22 years in practice:

I do a general physical and take a history, including sex history. Hormones are sometimes indicated because the sex life dictates it, even when the Pap smear isn't low in hormones yet. Vaginal membranes can become dry and thin, making the sex experience painful. Also you can tell the need by looking at a woman's genitals.
I've always used the minimum dosage that was clinically helpful. And always guidance with it. That would be the equivalent of 0.625 mg Premarin. Then I lower that, if possible. Occasionally I go to 1.25 mg, but then I bring the patient in every three to six months and try to reduce the dose at that time.

I prescribe estrogen for five days out of each week because I think we're likely to avoid withdrawal bleeding, even though that hasn't been proven yet. The result is also better than other types of cycles because it is more regular. Some patients I treat with localized vaginal estrogen cream, not systemically at all.

Let me emphasize that if she doesn't need them, she does not get them at all. Otherwise, it is an individual thing. Some patients are on estrogen maintenance for years, others for a little while during menopause. A patient shouldn't stop suddenly though— that may cause withdrawal bleeding.

*How do you
determine the need
for hormones,
and the dosage?*

*What treatment
program do
you recommend?*

*How long
should therapy
be continued?*

[2]   DR. B (Female) Family Medicine, 16 years in practice:

I judge by symptoms. I pay more attention to the patient than the vaginal smear. And remember, lots of women aren't bothered by symptoms at all.

I used to start at the equivalent of 1.25 mg Premarin as a beginning dose. Now I will start at 0.625 mg and explain that it appears that the risk of developing endometrial cancer increases in patients who take large doses of estrogen for a long time. As a result, we don't give as much nor give it for as long a period as we used to.

I use the cycle of three weeks of estrogen and one week off. I don't add the second hormone (progestin). It has the effect of withdrawing the contents of the uterus, but most women don't want to start periods again.

Last year I changed women over fifty from birth control pills to Premarin or its equivalent. I still use the esrogen, but I educate the patient more and let her make up her mind as to whether she wants to take it.

After six or eight months of being on estrogen, I suggest she take a month's rest to see how she feels. If she's still getting symptoms, she can go back on again. I give a prescription for one year and then insist she come in again for a pelvic and Pap smear. If there has been any unusual bleeding, I do a biopsy to see what's going on.

[3]   DR. C (Male) Family Medicine, 12 years in practice:

Only rarely would I recommend hormone therapy at all. It must be done very carefully because it is interfering with nature. Before a patient starts, she should look into it as extensively as possible, then make a decision with the advice of a doctor. If a woman decides she wants estrogen, I would prescribe the lowest dosage possible.

I would recommend any safeguards I could think of against the side effects. Estrogens cause vitamin deficiencies. A person would have to take a full range of vitamins and minerals to make up for what is lost. That in itself should give a woman pause before she starts taking estrogen.

For as short a time as possible.

42

*How do you
determine the need
for hormones,
and the dosage?*

*What treatment
program do
you recommend?*

*How long
should therapy
be continued?*

[4]   DR. D (Female) Gynecologist, 25 years in practice:

By her symptoms. I believe the need often varies with an individual's activity. Women in competitive occupations, required a great deal of energy, probably need a higher level of estrogen than those who lead quieter lives. Stress increases the number of flushes and sweats. Women are more apt to have physical problems when they are pushing themselves.
I prescribe just enough to control symptoms.

I prescribe estrogen cyclically — three weeks on with one week off. Some doctors add a progestin during the third week as a precaution against a build-up of the endometrium. But then withdrawal bleeding may occur, and some women have painful or profuse periods. Most don't like to be bothered with periods, especially in their sixties or seventies.

It varies, depending upon the patient. Some women get the symptoms back as soon as they go off. Others find they can get along well without hormones after awhile.

[5]   DR. E (Female) Gynecologist, 10 years in practice:

I judge by specific symptoms. Hot flushes and vaginal drying are the only symptoms which are consistently relieved by estrogens.
I usually start on a low-medium dosage, and if this isn't effective in relieving the hot flushes, then I'd increase the dosage. If she complains of breast tenderness, as some women do, I'd decrease the dosage.

I prescribe that hormones be omitted for five days at the beginning of each month. For women who have a uterus, I prescribe Provera (progestin) for five days at the end of the cycle each month or sometimes every three months, depending upon each individual case. She may have a period if the uterine lining is getting at all built up, but many don't bleed at all.

I usually keep women on through age sixty or sixty-five, then decrease the dose gradually. Now this is different from the old idea of "estrogen forever," when women were loaded with high doses of estrogen, with no cyclic system at all, with the promise of keeping young forever.

*How do you
determine the need
for hormones,
and the dosage?*

*What treatment
program do
you recommend?*

*How long
should therapy
be continued?*

[6]   DR. F (Male) Gynecologist, 20 years in practice:

I am a believer in the use of postmenopausal hormones for most women. Any time a woman develops symptoms of a hormone lack or shows up with a low estrogen index on her Pap smear, it's probably time for her to start taking hormones. The vagina and cervix are more sensitive to estrogen than any other tissue, so even in the absence of other symptoms, if I see a low estrogen level in the smear, I'll start the patient on a hormone replacement program.

I've done the dosage rather arbitrarily. I think the woman entering into this phase usually needs more estrogen to control her symptoms than she will five years later. I usually use the equivalent of 1.25 mp Premarin, then at about fifty-five years reduce that dose by one-half.

I prescribe estrogen for three weks at a time and add 5 mg of Provera (progestin) to it the last five days. Then when I reduce the dose at fifty-five years, try to go to an eight-week cycle, adding Provera the seventh week. Not all women—only about one-half of them—will have bleeding. That means the lining of the uterus has not built up enough to slough off.

I believe a woman should continue a maintenance dose of hormones indefinitely. If you use estrogen as a stop-gap measure to relieve symptoms for a short time, as some are advocating now, you probably should not prescribe them at all. It should be easier for a woman to get over symptoms at fifty than at sixty-five. Of course, if a woman has had a hysterectomy, there's no worry about the lining build-up. That might be one offshoot of this controversy, the easing of the rules regulating when hysterectomies can be performed. I would not go so far as to advocate a hysterectomy for a menopausal woman as a preventative measure, but I will be performing more office biopsies to check on what is going on in the uterus of postmenopausal patients. The disadvantage to that procedure now is the expense, but as the technique is used more, the cost should go down.

44

How do you
determine the need
for hormones,
and the dosage?

What treatment
program do
you recommend?

How long
should therapy
be continued?

[7] DR. G (Male) Endocrinologist, 25 years in practice:

Every woman over fifty is estrogen-deficient by the standards of a thirty-year-old. It is an accident of evolution that the ovaries gradually fail, so I try to give what would be a maintenance dose for a woman of thirty, equivalent to the dosage of birth control pills. If a patient is uncomfortable with that much, I cut her down to a smaller dosage and hope it will do her some good. It is tough to measure estrogen levels. There are effective tests, but they are expensive. I disagree with many on the value of the vaginal smear—it is practically useless. It is better to measure the FSH (follicle stimulating hormone secreted by the pituitary gland) levels in the blood. A full dose of estrogen will bring the FSH levels down to normal.

My patients take estrogen every day except the first week of every month, then add Provera (progestin) the last week of every month. So she is off both of them for that first week. This cyclic program does mimic nature. An alternative would be to induce a period once or twice a year. If a patient takes a full dose of estrogen and progestin for two weeks, she will have a period. You could call this a medical D and C. Now this is speculation, but I think such a treatment would protect her from this possible cancerous condition. The techniques now available by which gynecologists can do endometrial biopsies when they do Pap smears should also help to take care of that problem.

She should continue the therapy indefinitely unless there are side effects. Estrogen slows down one aspect of the aging process.

In contrast to the striking differences of opinion expressed in these interviews, there were some points all the doctors agreed upon.

Most important—any unexpected vaginal bleeding or even spotting should be investigated immediately by a doctor. One of our correspondents asked that we make this point emphatically because of her own experience. A biopsy revealed she had developed an endometrial cancer. "And all I had noticed was just a few tiny spots of blood. If it hadn't been for all this publicity, I would certainly have ignored the symptoms."

The interviewees also agreed that women who had had breast or uterine cancer or a history of thromboembolic disease (blood clots) should not take estrogen.

They also all agreed about the benefits of the therapy. Estrogen does alleviate the two main menopausal symptoms of hot flushes and vaginal dryness. Some believe that estrogen probably also helps to prevent osteoporosis (thinning of bones) and cardiovascular disease. Two of the doctors spoke of the patient's general sense of well-being under estrogen therapy. One reported that women will come back and say, "What was in those pills you gave me? I feel like a new person."

Besides the specific information gained from these interviews, we also received an important general impression of the essential objectivity of the scientific mind. It is a quality which is both chilling and comforting. Chilling because these medical professionals can weigh so dispassionately the possible risks of treatment programs with little apparent concern about the anguish that an individual patient might suffer. The two of us who conducted the interviews often found ourselves, as middle-aged women confronting these questions for ourselves as well as our readers, exchanging glances of distress as our interviewees launched forth enthusiastically upon their recitals of theories and statistics. The doctors seemed to feel challenged by all these uncertainties. We were dismayed.

At the same time, we decided we should probably feel reassured that medical researchers can proceed upon their logical analyses of these complicated problems, untouched by emotional distractions. We also found ourselves peculiarly awed by the realization that each of us lives in a body so remarkably complex that even after all these years of investigation, so much is still shrouded in mystery.

Are there other dangers in hormone therapy?

Less than two months after we had completed these interviews, another disturbing study was reported in *The New England Journal of Medicine* (August 19, 1976). This one, a joint study by the Harvard School of Public Health, the National Cancer Institute, and the University of Louisville School of Medicine, suggested a possible association between menopausal estrogen therapy and an increased risk of breast cancer. Of the 1891 women who were followed for twelve years, 49 developed breast cancer. In the general population 39.1 would have been expected to develop the disease. The authors themselves cautioned that the number of women studied was limited. They did agree, however, that estrogen does not offer women protection against breast cancer, as had been claimed by some doctors in the past.

In an effort to keep our information up-to-date, we wrote to eight of the doctors we had interviewed (the ninth had been reluctant to prescribe estrogen under any circumstances), asking whether this new evidence had changed their minds about estrogen therapy. None of them said they would change their procedures on the basis of that report. One criticized the method of research, asking why the doctors had not also studied a control group of women who had not taken estrogen with which to compare the cases cited. He also pointed out that in the "general population" to which these patients had been compared, a substantial number would also have taken estrogen.

Another of our interviewees sent some material, quoting statements from other doctors who deplore the overreaction to all these anti-estrogen studies. One of them, Dr. Felix Rutledge, President of the Oncology Society of America, speaking at the organization's fifty-eighth annual meeting, is reported to have said that "journalistic sensationalism and Food and Drug Administration proclamations have frightened women into premature action and placed an unnecessary burden on physicians to explain their practice." Dr. Rutledge did recommend, however, that the amounts of hormones prescribed should be kept small and administered only to selected patients, who should be monitored regularly.

Among the FDA "proclamations" was a press release on September 27, 1976, announcing that the FDA had ordered revisions of estrogen labeling for physicians' use and had proposed that a special brochure, in lay language, be provided women at the time they purchase the medication.

Dr. Alexander Schmidt, Commissioner of Food and Drugs, said, "Estrogens are valuable drugs. They are needed when the symptoms of the 'change of life' become severe. FDA's purpose is to keep these drugs on the market but to reduce overuse and misuse. Because these drugs can cause harm as well as good and because they are different from many other drugs in that they are given to healthy women undergoing the natural process of menopause, the FDA believes it essential that women be informed and that they decide for themselves if the risks are worth the benefits."

Among the points emphasized in both the patients' brochure and the doctors' pamphlet are these:

☐ It is important that if women take estrogens they take them in the lowest possible dose that will control symptoms and only as long as the drug is needed. Physicians should re-evaluate the need for continuing estrogen treatment at least every six months.

☐ Women should be examined by their physician no less than once every six months while taking estrogens.

☐ Pregnant women should never be given estrogens. Estrogens may damage the offspring.

☐ In general, estrogens should not be taken by women with breast or uterine cancer, undiagnosed abnormal vaginal bleeding, clotting in the legs or lungs, or by women who have had heart disease, angina (chest pains), a stroke, or gall bladder disease.

☐ Estrogens should not be used to treat simple nervousness during menopause, because they have not been shown to be effective for that purpose. Neither have estrogens been shown to keep the skin soft or to keep women feeling young.

Judging from this, it would seem that the current trend in the FDA coincides with the policy feminists have been advocating for several years—give women the facts regarding their health care and let them make up their own minds.

4

How Was Hormone Therapy Developed?

*Why haven't doctors known about the
dangers in hormone therapy long before
this? They've been prescribing
them for years, haven't they?*
From a letter to *Women in Midstream*

Another way to assess the present state of medical knowledge about the treatment of menopause is to look back—not so many years—to the beginnings of hormone therapy.

Recognizing how males have dominated the medical profession, it should come as no surprise that the earliest interest in hormone replacement therapy grew out of efforts to rejuvenate aging men's waning sexual powers. As early as 1889, a French physiologist, Brown-Sequard, reported to the Societé de Biologie in Paris that he had injected himself with the extracts from animals' testicles and had experienced "renewed physical strength and an invigoration of cerebral function." The Societé rejected his findings as being too subjective, but his techniques for producing glandular extracts were subsequently adopted as guides for later experiments.

Two men in the nineteenth century did try to relieve females' problems. In 1893 another French scientist, Regis de Bordeaux, used an ovarian extract injection to treat a patient for "insanity" following a surgically induced menopause. And in 1896 a German doctor, Theodore Landau, used desiccated ovaries for the treatment of menopausal symptoms, with apparently inconclusive results.

Then this type of experimentation lagged for several years. Writing in 1922 in *Endocrinology*, Dr. Emil Novak observed that there had been no "noteworthy advance in ovarian therapy in the quarter century since Landau had reported upon his methods."

Other methods of glandular therapy had caused excitement in the intervening years, however. The two most colorful came to be known as the Voronoff and Steinach methods, each named after its creator.

Dr. Serge Voronoff was a flamboyant Russian surgeon who traveled widely, publicizing the wonders of his technique. He was the developer of the renowned "monkey-gland operation," in which the sex glands of chimpanzees were implanted in human males. Several of his rejuvenated elderly patients readily testified to the wondrous results of the transplants.

By 1924 Voronoff had adapted the technique to the treatment of women, by implanting in them youthful ovaries from female chimpanzees. In a book he published in 1928, the doctor told about one case of "high moral value." A forty-eight-year-old Brazilian woman had come to him for rejuvenation because her husband had left her, finding her too old and fat. After the operation, the doctor wrote, "her muscles became firmer and her eyes glowed with the light of happiness." In fact, she was so thoroughly rejuvenated, she refused to return to her husband because "he did not deserve me," she said. Apparently many patients did report improved vigor, but the results were inevitably temporary as the body either absorbed or rejected the foreign implantations.

At this same time, a Viennese physiologist, Professor Eugen Steinach, approached the problem of male rejuvenation from an entirely different direction. He theorized that a male's sex glands could be stimulated to produce more hormones if their second function of producing spermatozoa were eliminated. So his treatment involved an early type of vasectomy in which the spermal duct was tied off.

Steinach also adapted his technique to the treatment of women. Their glands, the ovaries included, were "activated" through X-ray treatments. This procedure created particular excitement among women when a popular novelist of the day, Gertrude Atherton, publicized the remarkable improvement she had enjoyed after undergoing a series of Steinach treatments. She said at first she suffered torpor, but then "I had the sensation of a black cloud lifting . . . my brain seemed sparkling with light."

"Women from all over the English-speaking world wrote to me to inquire about the treatment," she later reported in her autobiography. At the same time, Mrs. Atherton wrote, she was "denounced from the pulpit, and certain club women, who regarded anything beyond their limited comprehension as immoral, banded together in an endeavor to stop this book before it should have contaminated the virtuous American public."

We would thank those club women for their opposition today, when the dangers of X-ray radiation are more clearly understood. The Steinach treatment for females would be rejected not only for its questionable hypothesis of reactivation of glands, but, more importantly, for its potentially devastating effects upon internal organs.

Another rejuvenation method which became popular in the 1920s and '30s was called *organotherapy*. It consisted of the ingestion of pills made from the organs of various animals. Scientists understood the importance of the endocrine glands, but had not perfected the techniques for extracting hormones. The ingredients of one such capsule were listed as:

thymus of calf	thyroid of sheep
ovaries of heifer	pancreas of pig
spleen of pig	orchitic juice of bull
duodenum of pig	veal liver
hypophysis of ox	prostate of pig
kidneys of ox	

Other medications were simpler. In 1929 a Dr. H. Jaworski was quoted in *The Literary Digest* as having claimed that the ingestion of active serum from a bull had proved effective for both men and women in combatting aging. However, he believed that the ingestion of young human blood plasma worked even better as a regenerator.

Such versions of organotherapy were received with special enthusiasm by women suffering menopausal discomforts. In *American Medicine* (November 1933), Dr. Herman F. Strongin wrote, "The educational propaganda, especially that dealing with gland therapy which has caught the fancy of many women in the 4th and 5th decades of life, is unfortunately being spread with ingenuous piquancy by some reputable newspapers and magazines whose reading public is comprised of women."

But as knowledge of the female reproductive glands and their secretions advanced, the direction of hormonal therapy for women changed. By 1926 Drs. Edgar Allen and Jean Paul Pratt had published in the *Journal of the American Medical Association* their proof that female sex hormones regulate menstruation. In 1929 Dr. Edward A. Doisy and his associates announced that, working with the urine from pregnant females, they had isolated and crystallized a female hormone which they called *theelin.* later named *estrone.* About the same time, Dr. Willard Allen isolated and crystallized *progesterone*, the second type of female hormone.

In 1932 Drs. Samuel Geist and Frank Spielman described in the *American Journal of Obstetrics and Gynecology* some successes in treating menopausal patients with theelin (estrone). "The premise that menopause symptoms are associated with a cessation of ovarian function is both reasonable and logical," they wrote. "[Our] statistical study would appear to justify the conclusion of the existence of an efficacious hormonal preparation useful in menopause. . . . Studies by other observers on this and similar preparations have almost invariably resulted in favorable reports."

These early treatments consisted of injections of hormonal solutions or sometimes implantations of crystallized hormones beneath the skin of the thigh or abdomen. The second method was considered beneficial because the effects were longer lasting than the injections. Both treatments were expensive, however, and the supplies of hormones limited because they were derived from human sources.

But these problems were solved in 1936 when two Pennsylvania State College researchers, Russell E. Marker and Thomas S. Oakwood, made a synthetic form of estrogen. This opened the way for the manufacture of a cheaper and more potent hormone-like substance which could be made available to all women who needed it. It also made the eventual development of an oral contraceptive pill possible.

Another big step in hormone therapy occurred in the early 1940s when James R. Goodall of McGill University developed an estrogen extract from pregnant mares' urine. Termed *conjugated equine estrogen*, it is about half as potent as synthetic estrogens, but seems to create fewer unpleasant side effects for many women. Though there are other brands of this type on the market today, Premarin, from Ayerst Laboratories, is by far the most widely used in this country.

A review of popular magazines of the 1940s and '50s reflects the enthusiasm with which hormone therapy was adopted, especially for menopausal symptoms. *Business Week* in September 1943 reported on the "Hormone Profits" being realized through the marketing of pregnant mares' urine. In December 1945 the same magazine reviewed the legal battle raging between Schering Laboratory and Glidden Paints because the paint company wanted the right to produce progesterone from soybean by-products, but Schering held a patent on its production. *Newsweek* of June 18, 1954 quoted Dr. E. Kost Shelton, a UCLA geriatrician, as advising the use of estrogen not only during the menopause, but well into the aging years.

In the 1960s several endocrinologists, under the influence of Dr. Robert A. Wilson and the Wilson Research Foundation, began to advocate a hormone treatment program in which the patient regularly adds progesterone to her cycle of estrogen to induce the shedding of the uterine lining as a safeguard against the build-up of tissue in which cancer might develop. Though Dr. Wilson touted his system of therapy rather over-enthusiastically in his popular book *Feminine Forever*, his theories were also published in professional journals, and he became an influential pioneer in this type of treatment.

Why wasn't more attention paid to early warnings?

Even as the promise of female hormone therapy was being widely publicized, some researchers were advising caution. As early as 1936 the *American Journal of Obstetrics and Gynecology* included an article by Drs. Emil Novak and Enmei Yui which warned that estrogen therapy might cause a build-up of endometrial tissue under estrogenic stimulation. "This seems significant," they wrote, "in view of the growing opinion that the carcinogenic possibilities of estrogenic substances are most to be reckoned with in those organs in whose growth and activities estrogen normally plays an important part" (i.e., the cervix, uterus, and breasts). In January 1940 the American Medical Association announced that synthetic hormones might be potentially dangerous, possibly contributing to liver damage or cancer.

And in December 1947 Dr. S. B. Gusberg wrote in the *American Journal of Obstetrics and Gynecology*, "Another human experiment has been set up in recent years by the widespread administration of estrogens to postmenopausal women. The relatively low cost of stilbestrol (synthetic estrogen) and the ease of its administration have made its general use promiscuous. Uterine bleeding provoked in postmenopausal patients by this medication has become such a commonplace occurrence that an idiomatic expression 'stilbestrol bleeding' has found use."

Why wasn't more attention paid to these early warnings? One doctor we put the question to said some of the study methods were considered at the time to be scientifically inadequate. Others were based upon animal experiments which were not applicable to humans. And, finally, he speculated that many doctors probably hated to give up a treatment which had proved to be so effective.

This latter sentiment was expressed by Dr. Samuel H. Geist when he wrote in 1941, "... it is suggested that extreme caution be used before attributing carcinogenic properties to estrogen in human beings, lest an extremely valuable therapeutic agent be condemned unjustly."

The most disturbing question to the lay person is what part drug companies have played in promoting their products. Medical journals are filled with advertisements praising the benefits of all kinds of hormone pills. And we understand that drug salesmen push their wares like high-pressure lobbyists. But our most disquieting discovery has been that much of the research on menopause treatment has been subsidized by the medical laboratories which manufacture hormones. How objective can such work be? It is a question we cannot resolve here. But it is one for which a skeptical consumer must demand answers.

What should a woman do about her own menopausal symptoms?

First, be alert to the advances in knowledge and technology which doctors have promised, probably within the next five years. Among the developments to watch for should be: simpler procedures for office biopsies to check on the condition of the uterus, simpler accurate tests for an individual's hormone levels, additional knowledge about the types of estrogens and progestins most suitable for therapy, and more information about estrogen's functions so that the benefits of hormone therapy may be more accurately weighed against its risks.

Medical journals (sometimes available in public libraries) are usually pretty hard to understand, but popular news and women's magazines include quite comprehensive, and usually reliable, reports on medical developments. Whatever the source of information, no one should ever hesitate to check out any question with her doctor if it seems relevant to her condition.

In the meantime we believe each person should consider her own state of health and medical history. She should weigh the risks she is willing to take against the benefits she will enjoy. Among the women we hear from at the YWCA, the attitudes toward hormone therapy vary.

One told us recently, "I feel so much better taking estrogen. It seems to relieve my aching bones and muscles. I'm going to keep on taking it. I'll keep the dose as small as possible and check with my doctor more often, though."

Another said she would keep on taking estrogen, mainly for hot flushes which keep her awake, but with the recent publicity about uterine cancer, she had agreed with her doctor that she should add a progestin at the end of each cycle. "I hate to start hassling with menstrual periods again, though," she grumbled.

We did not get much help when we asked the doctors we interviewed about alternatives to estrogen therapy. A few women told us they have been given other medications. Some have taken male hormones for the control of excessive bleeding, but they complain of irritating side effects. Others have tried Bellergal, a combination of belladonna and phenobarbital, for the alleviation of hot flushes, but it could be habit-forming. Others have been given tranquilizers and sleeping pills for nervous tension and insomnia, but most of the women we hear from are reluctant to depend upon drugs like these.

A number of women told us they have quit taking hormones altogether and are working out their own therapies, with their doctors' approval. One asked us to pass on the advice that a woman cut down gradually on estrogen pills, though. "I quit cold turkey," she said, "and felt pretty depressed for a couple of months. When I told my doctor, he said I should have tapered off by taking them every other day for awhile, then cutting down on the dosage. I'm doing O.K. now, but it took about six months for my body to adjust. So tell your readers to be patient."

Another reported she had been bothered by hot flushes only recently and had decided not to start on hormones. "I'm taking a multivitamin every day and exercising as often as I can to see if that will help. So far so good."

"I'm experimenting with relaxation techniques," one friend reported. "I figure if I have something definite to do when my nerves jangle or my face burns, I'll feel like I can control my body better."

Women cannot solve all these scientific puzzles. But perhaps they can prod the medical profession into doing the research required to answer them, by nagging their doctors with persistent questions and by fully reporting their symptoms and experiences. In short, they can take the initiative for their own well-being.

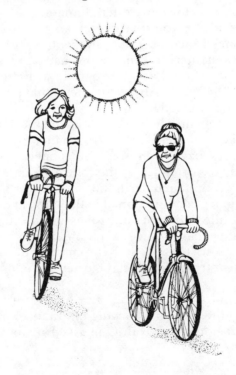

5
How Did Our Grandmothers Treat Menopause?

In my day women didn't pay much
attention to 'the change,' as we called it.
They just expected to suffer, if they
had any problems. It's natural, isn't it?
And it comes to everybody—'Judy
O'Grady and the Colonel's Lady'—as
my Irish grandmother used to say.
Keep your mind off yourself, that's
what I say.

Evelyn (78 years old)

"What did our grandmothers do? They didn't have any of these hormone pills, did they?" These questions have been asked of us so often that we decided to interview some post-menopausal women about their own experiences, and their mothers', if they could remember. The project wasn't easy. Most older women didn't want to talk about it. One said, "That was such a terrible time for me, I don't even want to think about it." Another scolded us, "I don't believe in talking about such things. It's not proper at all."

But the few interviews we succeeded in getting produced some revealing statements:

"My eighty-year-old aunt was visiting us when I first started having hot flushes at night. She had been a nurse, so I thought it would be all right to ask her advice. She said to put a bucket of ice water underneath my bed. That's what they used to do in her time. It didn't help me any though. Then I

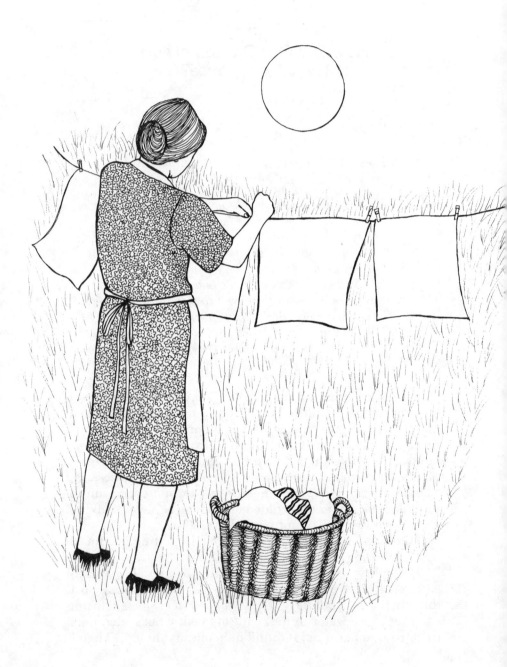

heard about hormones—they were just coming in. So I went to my doctor and he gave me some. They helped right away."

—Sarah (85 years old)

"I didn't have any problem with hot flushes or anything like that. But I would get so nervous. I'd work at the store all day, then come home so tired, but still couldn't rest. I used to go out at night and walk the streets. Whenever a big truck came by and nobody could hear, I'd stand there and scream and scream. That relieved my nerves some."

—Mildred (73 years old)

"I went through menopause at the same time my husband was very ill. I remember the doctor saying that it was too bad I had to face both things at the same time. He used to give me shots. 'To help my nerves,' he would say. I don't know what it was. Could it have been hormones then? I never even asked."

—Ellen (77 years old)

"I didn't have a bit of trouble. I'm from the old country, you know. Women over there didn't have that kind of trouble. We were awfully strong. And did we work hard. When I came to New York, I worked in a beauty shop and I was always surprised at the fuss American women made about the 'change.' One customer used to get so excited when she felt a hot flash, she'd put her head in our icebox. I'd tell her, 'Don't do that, you'll melt the ice.' "

—Gerta (80 years old)

"I didn't have much trouble myself, which surprised me because my mother suffered terribly. She was over forty when I was born, so I was still young and around the house a lot. She was so depressed. It scared me. She talked about dying a lot, though she lived a good many years longer. Poor Mother, she was so reserved. I'm sure she never talked with anybody about her fears."

—Maria (82 years old)

These comments piqued our curiosity so much that we decided to look back even further, into the late nineteenth and early twentieth centuries, by reviewing some publications from those times. With one notable exception, the popular books and magazines which we examined contained no explicit information about menopause.

Good Housekeeping Magazine for July 1912 did include one article which, at first glance, seemed promising. Entitled,

"Ordeals of the Middle-Aged Woman," it started out by quoting a "matron" who said, "I am nearing the dullest place in my life. I feel like furniture of the Victorian period. I have some of that and I hate it. Old furniture—a veritable antique—is a treasure while a new piece is up-to-date and in fashion, but furniture fifty years old is an atrocity, and so are people when they get near that age." But the author of the article, Virginia Terhune Van de Water, only cited this woman as a foolish example of an aging female, then went on to discuss all the satisfactions of growing old, without ever mentioning possible physical problems, certainly not menopause.

The single exception we found to this general reticence was a novel, *The Dangerous Age*, written by a Danish woman, Karin Michaelis, and translated into English in 1911. It tells the story of Elsie Lindtner, a well-bred woman in her early forties. In love with a younger man and wracked by unconsummated passions, she left her husband to live alone on an island. Her story unfolds through journals and letters. At one point she muses about her advancing years:

> Somebody should found a vast and cheerful sisterhood for women between forty and fifty; a kind of refuge for the victims of the years of transition. For during that time women would be happier in voluntary exile, or at any rate entirely separated from the other sex.
>
> Since all are suffering from the same trouble, they might help each other to make life, not only endurable, but harmonious. We are all more or less mad then, although we struggle to make others think us sane.

Even Karin Michaelis never used the word *menopause* in her novel, but the allusions to "the shadowy future" and "the years of transition" must have seemed daringly outspoken. Most women in those days would never have gone as far as that, especially in print. We did turn up a few scattered references in personal letters to what might have been menopausal discomforts. In writing to a friend about her mother, then fifty-two years old, Emily Dickinson said, "Mother has been an invalid since we came home. . . . Vinnie and I 'got settled,' and still we keep our Father's house, and Mother lies upon the lounge, or sits in her easy chair. I don't know what her sickness is, for I am but a simple child, and frightened at myself." Later in the year a family friend wrote, "Mrs. D's health is poor and she is at the water-cure in North Hampton" (a popular treatment for "female complaints" at that time).

Another reference that seems especially apt occurs in a letter by Susan Hale, a widely-traveled writer of her day. Writing to her sister from Matunuck, Rhode Island, in September 1886, she tells how relieved she was to see all the young people leave her vacation home at last: "There is a good deal of clatter and bang about running such a household, and I now feel like a fool, or a squeezed lemon, or a pricked balloon or any of these things." Whether or not this was intended as an allusion to menopausal fatigue — she was fifty-three at the time — her words describe the condition vividly.

Women in the nineteenth century were expected to be modest — even ignorant — about their bodily functions. When Dr. Edward H. Dixon explained such things in a book for women in 1847, he first justified his undertaking in the introduction:

> It is difficult to perceive either the force or propriety of the arguments used by those who allege that the diseases of woman form an improper subject for popular instruction. From her position in the social scale, she is subjected to so many causes of physical degeneration from the evident design of nature — as proved by the rare examples of perfection in her sex now and then seen — that it seems but an act of humanity to make an effort for her instruction in some of the more common evils that so constantly beset her.

The reader of Dr. Dixon's book was also reassured by a quotation from a Boston newspaper printed on the fly leaf: "In communicating the necessary information to avoid ministering to impure feelings, to use no expression that could raise a blush on the most delicate cheek, to write no word that could cause the most careful mother to withhold the book from her daughter of suitable age, certainly required a nice judgment and great caution. We believe that this work combines all these requisites. *Boston Chronotype*."

Another doctor of that time, Charles D. Meigs, Professor of Midwifery and the Diseases of Women and Children at the Jefferson Medical College, Philadelphia, saw a danger in women's modesty about their bodiy ills. In his widely used medical textbook, *Woman: Her Diseases and Remedies*, he wrote, "The relations between the sexes are of so delicate a character, that the duties of a medical practitioner are necessarily more difficult, when he comes to take charge of a patient laboring under any one of the great host of female complaints. . . . So great, indeed, is the embarrassment arising from fastidiuosness on the part either of the female herself, or of the practitioner, or both, that, I am persuaded, much of the ill success of treatment may be justly charged thereto."

But Dr. Meigs also expressed some admiration for this fastidiousness: "I confess I am proud to say, that, in this country generally . . . women prefer to suffer the extremity of danger and pain rather than waive those scruples of delicacy which prevent their maladies from being fully explored. I think this is an evidence of the presence of a fine morality in our society; but nevertheless, it is true that a greater candor on the part of the patient, and a more resolute and careful inquiry on that of the practitioner, would scarcely fail to bring to light, in their early stages, the curable maladies which, by faults on both sides, are now misunderstood, because concealed, and, consequently, mismanaged and rendered at last incurable."

The "greater candor" should exist only between a doctor and his patient, however. Dr. Meigs deplored the newspaper advertisements which depicted women wearing such devices as "utero-abdominal supporters." "Who wants to know, or who ought to know that the ladies have abdomens and wombs but us doctors?" he asks. "When I was young, a woman had no legs even, but only feet, and possibly *ankles*; now, forsooth, they have utero-abdominal supporters, not in fact only, but in the very newspapers."

Is it any wonder that midnineteenth century women tried to avoid doctors with attitudes like these? At least one book explicitly encouraged such distrust. In *Letters to the People on Health and Happiness*, Catharine Beecher reported shocking experiences which women had endured at the hands of medical practitioners. The delicacy with which she discussed the subject, necessarily leaving much to the imagination, made her descriptions thoroughly frightening: "During the later periods of my investigations in regard to health," she wrote, "I became aware, not only of the general decay of the health of my own sex, but of the terrible suffering, both physical and mental, produced by internal organic displacements, resulting chiefly from a general debility of constitution. . . . In multitudes of cases, there was no possible remedy for this appalling evil but such daily *mechanical operations, both external and internal . . .* and that this was in most cases performed with bolted doors and curtained windows, and with no one present but patient and operator, there was a painful apprehension of evils."

One consequence of such apprehension is described in the autobiography of Elizabeth Blackwell, one of the first female doctors in the United States. (She was admitted to Geneva University Medical School in New York in 1847.) She tells about a friend, dying from a female disease "of a delicate nature," who urged Elizabeth to become a doctor, saying, "If I could have been treated by a lady doctor, my worst sufferings would have been spared me."

What woman wouldn't take her chances with a "uteroabdominal supporter" she saw advertised in a daily paper rather than risk the terrors hinted at by Miss Beecher?

According to the evidence reported in her book, the health of American females—young and old—was delicate. "The *standard of health* among American women is so low that few have a correct idea of *what a healthy woman is,*" she wrote. "I have again and again been told by ladies that they were 'perfectly healthy,' who yet, on close inquiry, would allow that they were subject to frequent attacks of neuralgia, or to periodic nervous headaches, or to local ailments, to which they had become so accustomed, that they were counted as 'nothing at all.' A woman who has tolerable health finds herself so much above the great mass of her friends in this respect, that she feels herself a prodigy of good health."

Twenty years later, apparently women's health had not improved much. Dr. Edward H. Clarke, Professor of Medicine at Harvard College, wrote in *Sex in Education*, "The delicate bloom, early but rapidly fading beauty, and singular pallor of American girls and women have almost passed into proverb. The first observation of a European that lands upon our shores is, that our women are a feeble race."

Today Dr. Clarke's argument that a major cause of this weakness was the demands put upon American young women in coeducational schools would be rejected out of hand. But when one considers the numerous children that most women bore, the hazards of childbirth, the high rate of infant mortality, not to mention the ravages of diseases like tuberculosis, smallpox, and pneumonia, it is little wonder that females may have seemed a "feeble race."

And if a woman lived through those hazards to reach menopause, the attitudes toward her condition then, and the treatments which the medical profession advised, offered little to comfort her.

For example, a French doctor, Colombat De L'Isere, whose medical book, *A Treatise on the Diseases and Special Hygiene of Females*, was translated into English by Dr. Meigs in 1850, mourned a woman's lost charms at the "critical age," the "turn of life." "She now resembles a dethroned queen, or rather a goddess whose adorers no longer frequent her shrine," he wrote. "Should she still retain a few courtiers, she can only attract them by the charm of her wit and the force of her talents." But he added, "In spite of the loss of all her physical advantages, the aged woman who is endowed with sense and wit, and who renounces all vain pretensions, and lays aside all coquetry, finds it in her power, by numerous admirable qualities, to become more worthy than ever of the warmest friendship and confidence of the male, whose lover she is not, but to whom she proves a sincere and consolatory friend."

Dr. Meigs, influenced, no doubt, by this French specialist, later wrote in his own textbook, "There is something melancholy in the conviction, that must attend the final cessation of the menses, of a decadence of the constitution. The subject of such a conviction is compelled to admit that she has now become—what? an old woman! . . . The pearls of the mouth are become tarnished—the haylike odor of the breath is gone, the rose has vanished from the cheek, and the lily is no longer the vain rival of the forehead or the neck. The dance is preposterous, and the throat no longer emulates the voice of the nightingale."

In contrast to these male experts' opinions, there is evidence that some women took a more positive view toward this "turn of life." Carroll Smith-Rosenberg, in an essay on women's health care in the nineteenth century quotes two women who reflected such attitudes. The first, Elizabeth Drinker, described by Professor Smith-Rosenberg as "a conservative and socially prominent Philadelphia Quaker," recorded in her diary (October, 1799) a conversation she had had with her daughter about the impending birth of yet another baby on her thirty-eighth birthday: "She is in pain at times, forerunning pains of a lingering labour, a little low spirited, poor dear Child. . . . I endeavoured to talk her into better Spirits, told her that the time of her birth was over by some hours, she was now in her 39th year, and that this might possibly be the last trial of this sort, if she could suckle her baby for two years to come, as she had several times done heretofore."

Freedom from pregnancy and the pains and hazards of childbirth was no small blessing for women in those days of ignorance about contraception.

The second statement comes from Eliza Farnham, a social reformer and women's suffrage advocate, who wrote in 1864 in *Woman and Her Era*, 'My acquaintance with women of the nobler sort has convinced me that many a woman has experienced, at times, a secret joy in her advancing age."

Describing herself as "having passed through the experience," Eliza Farnham called the postmenopausal years "a more exalted department of life." She added, "Let the idea . . . go abroad among the sex, that feminine life is divided by Nature into three periods (ante-maternal, maternal, and post-maternal), each of which is an advance . . . and we shall soon cease the wailing and lamentation over the first gray hair and the first wrinkle at the eyes."

The menopausal symptoms nineteenth-century doctors tried to alleviate were the same we are still familiar with today, but their methods would seem quaint, and often dangerous to twentieth-century patients. Extracting blood, either with leeches or by "cupping," was generally recommended for the treatment of hot flushes. The theory was not that the stopping of the menstrual flow allowed poisons to accumulate, as many women feared. Rather, that the cessation of the menses "must probably be the cause of considerable derangement in the circulation," as Dr. Dixon explained it in *Woman and Her Diseases*. But he reassured his readers that this condition could be relieved "by drawing a small quantity of blood from the arm."

An excessive flow during menstrual periods was often treated with cold water or ice packs applied to the lower abdomen while the rest of the body was kept warm. Dr.

Dixon also suggested that if a person of "clear judgment and a cool head" were in attendance, a woman under this treatment might be given a tablespoon of brandy and water every ten or fifteen minutes to revive her until the doctor arrived.

Dr. John C. Gunn, the author of *Domestic Medicine or the Poor Man's Friend in the Hours of Affliction, Pain, and Sickness,* recommended "purges of Epsom salts or castor oil . . . to cool the system" during a woman's "critical period." Or "if the pain in the womb be considerable," he suggested a woman might douche—"throw up the birth place"—with some cold slippery-elm water five or six times a day.

One treatment Dr. Gunn prescribed must have been pretty invigorating—the application of friction for one-half hour every morning and evening. The patient should rub her whole body, especially the limbs, with a brush or flannel. He claimed that this routine "kindles the natural warmth, promotes perspiration, opens the pores, and tends to dissipate stagnant humors." He did not mention what it did to the skin.

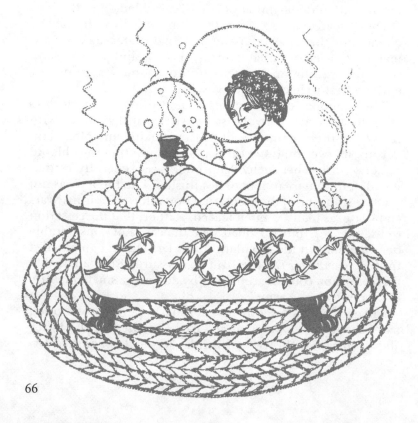

In a medical book translated from the German in 1910, *The Sexual Life of Woman In Its Physiological, Pathological and Hygienic Aspects*, Dr. E. Heinrich Kisch recommended water baths of various temperatures: A lukewarm bath for fifteen to twenty minutes would have a sedative effect upon the nervous system; a hot immersion bath of longer duration would increase the activity of the circulation through the skin; if an even more powerful effect were desired, a hot mineral bath was recommended. Only occasionally would a cold bath be indicated and then only for a very few minutes. This would counteract states of congestion and "bring about a general invigoration of the patient's nervous system." But cold sea-bathing was never recommended, "owing to its powerful refrigerative effect and the great mechanical influence of the moving water in the waves."

Some of the advice in these medical books still seems reasonable today. Menopausal women were encouraged to eat sensibly, exercise moderately, and get regular rest. But the details of treatment were decidedly restrictive. Dr. Colombat, for example, prohibited all tea, coffee, and spiritous liquors. For exercise he recommended housework because it provided the added pleasure of fulfilling one's duty. Riding in the country in the morning and caring for the "proper culture of flowers" would be beneficial too.

But Dr. Colombat was most definite in emphasizing the dangers of sleeping upon a feather bed. This practice, he warned, could promote plethoric accumulations, uterine hemorrhage, and constipation of the bowels. And, most hazardous of all, feather beds might "excite the generative organs, which should henceforth be left, as far as possible, in a state of inaction." A woman should, at this age, he added, "avoid all such circumstances as might tend to awaken any erotic thoughts in the mind, and reanimate a sentiment that ought rather to become extinct, such as the spectacle of lascivious figures, the reading of passionate novels, and, in fine, every thing calculated to cause regret for charms that are lost, and enjoyments that are ended for ever."

With medical advice like that, is it surprising that thousands of women turned to home remedies and health tonics to help themselves?

Like *Dr. Pierce's Favorite Prescription*, as advertised in *The Chicago-Herald*, September 14, 1901: "It makes weak women strong, sick women well." Not only that, Dr. Pierce also

GIVE HER A CHANCE

County President W.C.T.U., Mrs.
H.F. Roberts, of Kansas City,

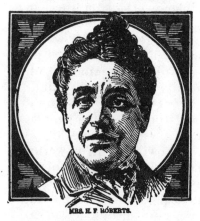

MRS. H. F. ROBERTS.

Says to All Sick Women:
"Give Mrs. Pinkham a Chance—
I Know She Can Help You
as She Did Me."

"DEAR MISS PINKHAM—The world
praises great reformers; their names and
fames are in the ears of everybody,
and the public press helps spread the
good tidings. Among them all Lydia E.
Pinkham's name goes to posterity with
a softly breathed blessing from the lips
of thousands upon thousands of women
who have been restored to their families when life hung by a thread, and by
thousands of others whose weary,
aching limbs you have quickened and
whose pains you have taken away"

AN OPEN LETTER

Addressed to Women
by the Treasurer of
the W.C.T.U. of Kansas City,
Mrs. E.C. Smith

"MY DEAR SISTERS:—I believe in
advocating and upholding everything that
will lift up and help women, and but
little use appears all knowledge and learning if you have not the health to enjoy it.

"Having found by personal experience
that Lydia E. Pinkham's Vegetable Compound is a medicine of rare virtue, and
having seen dozens of cures where my
suffering sisters have been dragged back
to life and usefulness from an untimely
grave simply by the use of a few bottles
of that Compound, I must proclaim its
virtues, or I should not be doing my duty
to suffering mothers and dragged-out
housekeepers.

"Dear Sister, is your health poor, do
you feel worn out and used up, especially
do you have any of the troubles which
beset our sex, take my advice; let the
doctors alone, try Lydia E. Pinkham's
Vegetable Compound; it is better than
any and all doctors, for it *cures*, and
they do not."—Mrs. E.C. Smith, 1919 Oak
St., Treasurer W.C.T.U., Kansas City, Mo.

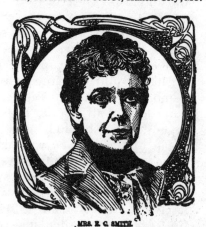

MRS. E. C. SMITH.

The compound that "restores natural cheerfulness, destroys despondency,
cures the great forerunner of serious trouble and relieves backache" was
advertised in this manner. Above, two endorsements by temperance workers.
At right, Pinkham advertising in a lighter mood.

invited women to consult him by letter, free of charge. "In his thirty years and over of medical practice," the ad read, "Dr. Pierce, assisted by his staff of nearly a score of physicians, had treated and cured more than half a million women."

Of course, the most famous home remedy of them all was *Lydia E. Pinkham's Vegetable Compound*. Except for the medical writers, she was the only one to refer openly to menopause. One of her ads reads: "There is no period in a woman's career which she approaches with so much anxiety as the 'change of life.' It is surprising what happy changes LYDIA E. PINKHAM'S VEGETABLE COMPOUND brings about in this condition. So marked is its power that all the trying days of the Change may be passed over in perfect safety. Women who have been dreading the Change, who have been taught to look upon it as something horrible, may now lay all such anxiety aside. Thousands of letters from women tell me that their life of distress and sleeplessness was changed to one of perfect comfort almost immediately."

It is easy to laugh at Lydia Pinkham from our perspective. Her advertisements, which always bore her smiling face, promised so much: "Sickness is often just as unnecessary as crime. Abide by the simple laws of nature, and doctors will seek other occupations. Just as there are reformatories to lead the criminal back to paths of rectitude, there is also a reformatory for guiding erring footsteps back to health. This grand reformatory is Lydia E. Pinkham's Vegetable Compound, which is bringing the roses of health to the cheeks of erstwhile suffering women all over the world."

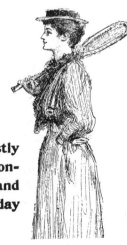

BEAUTY AT THE GRAND OPERA

The Women Admired by All.

Not Rich Wraps, Elegant and Costly Gowns, Expensive or Attractive Bonnets, but Perfect Forms, Features and Minds That Render Women of Today All Powerful.

Versions of Lydia songs and poems have proliferated over the years:

> Tell me, Lydia, of your secrets,
> And the wonders you perform,
> How you take the sick and ailing
> And restore them to the norm?
>
> Lizzie Smith had tired feelings,
> Terrible pains reduced her weight.
> She began to take the Compound,
> Now she weighs three hundred and eight.
>
> There's a baby in every bottle,
> So the old quotation ran.
> But the Federal Trade Commission
> Still insists you'll need a man.
>
> We'll sing of Lydia Pinkham
> And her love for the Human Race,
> How she sells her Vegetable Compound
> And the papers, they publish her face.

But Lydia Estes Pinkham was not just an unscrupulous hawker of her tonic. Born in 1819 in Lynn, Massachusetts, she was an early feminist and Abolitionist who also became interested in medical reform. When the Panic of 1873 wiped out the family's assets, they decided to start selling the health tonic she had been making and giving away to her neighbors for years. According to Jean Burton, one of her biographers, the evidence suggests that she sincerely believed in the claims made for her tonic. In later life she wrote booklets, which were distributed free upon request, describing in accurate scientific terms all aspects of female physiological development. As Jean Burton points out, it was the only thing of its kind available to women until the government started to issue such pamphlets.

In one way Lydia Pinkham's advertising was unusually honest. From the beginning she publicized the formula for her Compound:

8 oz. True Unicorn Root
8 oz. False Unicorn Root
6 oz. Life Root
6 oz. Black Cohosh
6 oz. Pleurisy Root
12 oz. Fenugreek Seed

Jean Burton explained the process: "Some were steeped, some soaked in cold water, some macerated in dilute alcohol. Then they were mixed all together and percolated through cloth, an operation like making fruit jellies. Before bottling, more alcohol ('used solely as a solvent and preservative') was added."

Doubtless the alcohol, measured at 18%, helped to soothe many nervous women, but perhaps we should pay special attention to these ingredients. According to Jean Burton, research conducted in the 1940s by government scientists, skeptical of the claims made for the tonic, indicated that it did reduce vasomotor disturbances (hot flushes) and helped to correct menstrual irregularities. Furthermore, the research showed that the Compound contained "hormonal factors." Apparently some of the plants in the formula, like many others that had been studied (among them, pussywillow, sarsaparilla, wild cherry, and yucca), contained "estrogenic materials, or principles capable of being converted into estrogen by chemical means."

So at a time when doctors were bleeding women to relieve menopausal symptoms, Lydia E. Pinkham, albeit unintentionally, was apparently providing them with an early-day version of hormone therapy.

Looking back, can we say that the treatments for menopause have improved in the later twentieth century? Women still complain about their medical care. And Geritol has replaced the Vegetable Compound for many. But certainly knowledge about the body has advanced. Now doctors understand about the importance of the endocrine glands and their hormones in the menopausal process. They no longer bleed women to "improve" their circulation. Some may argue, however, that the routine prescription of large doses of hormones may turn out to be just as questionable a practice. Readers in the twenty-first century may well look back with amusement at our ignorance.

One thing has improved, though. Women today feel more at ease with their bodies. And they are more willing to talk about their feelings and their experiences. The knowledge gained from this kind of communication will surely hasten our progress toward a fuller understanding.

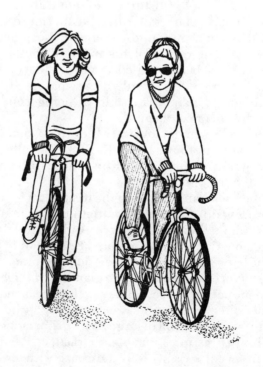

6
What Conditions May Require Surgery?

*My doctor says
I need a hysterectomy.
How do I know he isn't knife-happy?*
From a letter to
Women in Midstream

A few years ago Dr. Ralph Wright, a gynecologist, arguing in a professional journal for more liberalized attitudes toward elective hysterectomies, wrote, "The uterus has but one function: reproduction. After the last planned pregnancy, the uterus becomes a useless, bleeding, symptom-producing, potentially cancer-bearing organ and therefore should be removed."

He concluded the editorial by asking, "Will women in this modern era awaken to the fact that the monthly 'curse' is no longer a necessary part of life? Will there arise a crusader like Margaret Sanger? Or will the gynecologists with vision and courage take the lead and move to the logical conclusion? Perhaps both will occur. But regardless of the source of the final impetus, we will inevitably arrive. Elective hysterectomy is just around the corner."

Far from finding "crusaders" urging women to have their reproductive organs removed as early as possible, today women are being cautioned against unnecessary hysterectomies. Joann Rodgers, for example, a medical reporter for the Hearst Newspapers, cited these damning statistics in an article in the *New York Times Magazine* in September 1975:

- Hysterectomies are this nation's second most performed surgery—only tonsillectomies are more frequent.
- Hysterectomies are performed two and one-half times as often in the United States as in England and Wales, and four times as often as in Sweden.
- Hysterectomies are performed twice as often on patients with health insurance than on the uninsured.
- Hysterectomies will provide gynecologists in the United States with an estimated $400 million in fees in a single year.

Despite the suspicions aroused by statistics like these, there are times when a patient should have such surgery performed.

What is a hysterectomy?

First, to get the terminology straight, a *hysterectomy* means the removal of the uterus and cervix (the lower portion of the uterus). One often hears the expression "complete" hysterectomy as a description of the removal of the uterus, ovaries, and Fallopian tubes. But the medical term for removal of the ovaries is *oophorectomy* and of the tubes is *salpingectomy*. So if the uterus, Fallopian tubes, and both ovaries are removed, a patient has had a *hysterectomy* and *bilateral* (both sides) *salpingo-oophorectomy*.

Though it is unlikely that a doctor would use imprecise terminology, anyone faced with such surgery would be wise to clarify just what procedure the surgeon plans to follow. We have been surprised at the number of women we have encountered who are not at all sure what organs they did lose in their "complete" hysterectomies.

When is a hysterectomy necessary?

If a D and C (dilatation and curettage) has revealed cancerous cells in the uterus, there is no question that a hysterectomy should be performed. If such examination reveals abnormal cell changes, a doctor will usually recommend a hysterectomy as a preventative measure, especially if the patient is past the child-bearing age. The changes may not be malignant, but may be an indication of a "precancerous" condition.

If a fibroid tumor has increased in size or is causing troublesome bleeding, most doctors would recommend a hysterectomy. It is often possible to remove only the tumor, leaving the uterus intact. But for most women past the childbearing years this procedure would not seem very sensible.

Recently we talked with a woman in her sixties who had just had her uterus removed because of cancer in the lining. She was chiding herself because she had chosen to have only a fibroid tumor removed when she was forty-three, after having born four children. "If only I hadn't insisted upon keeping my uterus then, I wouldn't have had to go through all this surgery again," she said. "At the time it was all mixed up with preserving my femininity or some such feeling like that. I knew I didn't want more children."

If a woman experiences persistent heavy bleeding with no sign of a malignancy or abnormal cells, the necessity for a hysterectomy becomes less certain. We have heard opinions from both sides.

One correspondent wrote us, "I had suffered with very heavy periods for several years. I kept thinking pretty soon all this will dry up and go away. But by the time I reached fifty, I just got tired of the hassle and opted for a hysterectomy. And I'm so relieved now that I did it. I feel like a rejuvenated woman."

On the other hand, another friend in her fifties told us about her reluctance to accept her doctor's recommendation for a hysterectomy. "I gritted my teeth and simply told him I wanted another opinion. And you know what? The second doctor said he didn't think it was necessary. So I still have my uterus and am expecting those heavy periods to stop pretty soon."

In younger women (twenty-five to forty), a condition which sometimes requires surgery is endometriosis: here tissue like that which lines the uterus is found in other areas inside the abdomen, most frequently on the abdominal lining behind the uterus and on the surfaces of the ovaries.

Wherever it is growing, the tissue will then behave like the lining in the uterus, thickening and bleeding cyclically under the stimulus of the ovarian hormones. Endometriosis can sometimes cause severe problems, like infertility, abdominal discomfort, and painful intercourse.

In some cases, endometriosis can be treated with hormone therapy, usually a combination of estrogens and progestins. In others, limited surgery, to remove the overgrowths, may correct the condition. But sometimes, when the reproductive organs are widely involved, they must be removed altogether.

Because endometriosis develops during the fertile years, young women who undergo such surgery are plunged into menopause prematurely. Judging from the several letters we have received from these women, their symptoms are often unusually severe, probably because their bodies have not had the chance to slow down estrogen production gradually through natural aging. One woman described her surgical menopause as "devastating." Another said she was suffering from what might be called "withdrawal symptoms"—depression, nervousness, fatigue.

We always feel a special discouragement because we cannot offer better help to these women. Most of them are experimenting, under medical supervision, with different dosages of estrogens or combinations of estrogens and progestins. Some have decided to "tough it out" and wait for their bodies to adjust naturally to the altered hormone levels. Those who tell us occasionally that they do feel better after several months of adjustment provide the hopes for improvement which we can pass on to others.

Another quite common reason for a hysterectomy is a *prolapse*. Sometims if a woman's abdominal muscles and ligaments have lost their elasticity with age or through the stretching of several pregnancies, the abdominal organs will sag or drop down. This condition often creates pressure against the bladder, causing infections or stress incontinence—the involuntary leaking of a few drops of urine. This often happens when a person coughs or sneezes when her bladder is full.

The following sketch of the normal anatomical positions of the abdominal organs shows how these difficulties might develop when supporting muscles and ligaments relax.

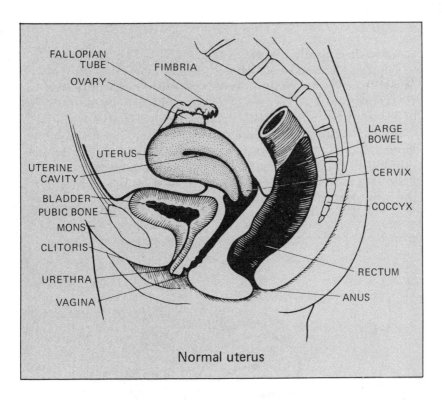

FALLOPIAN TUBE
FIMBRIA
OVARY
UTERUS
UTERINE CAVITY
BLADDER
PUBIC BONE
MONS
CLITORIS
URETHRA
VAGINA

LARGE BOWEL
CERVIX
COCCYX
RECTUM
ANUS

Normal uterus

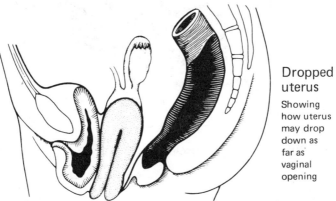

Dropped uterus

Showing how uterus may drop down as far as vaginal opening

If this condition becomes severe, it can cause difficulty with intercourse or discomfort with general pelvic congestion. If a woman is past child-bearing age, a surgeon will probably prefer to remove the uterus in correcting a prolapse. Then the vagina and other organs can be secured in their normal positions.

Can muscle relaxation be prevented?

There is an exercise which will help to maintain adequate muscle tone and perhaps prevent these prolapse conditions. It was originally advocated by Dr. Arnold Kegel as a means of correcting problems with urinary stress incontinence.

A muscle, called the *pubococcygeus*, extends from the pubic bone in front to the coccyx, or tail bone, in back. This muscle must be in good condition for normal bladder and rectal control. The following sketch shows its position in relation to the organs in the lower abdomen.

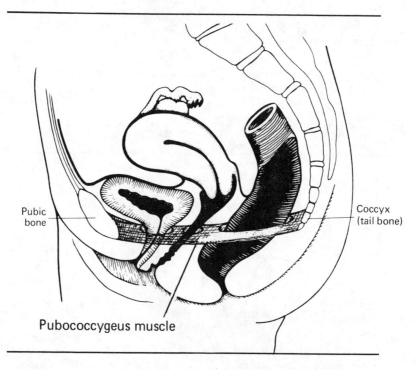

Pubic bone

Coccyx (tail bone)

Pubococcygeus muscle

The exercise involves contracting and relaxing this muscle many times a day. Dr. Kegel recommended that it be done three times a day for twenty minutes, for a total of three hundred contractions a day. Others have suggested it would be effective to do them several times a day, perhaps eight to ten per half hour, and up to two hundred.

One friend told us that she had noticed a marked improvement in just a few days with a minor problem she was having "leaking" when she sneezed or coughed. And she had done only about fifty contractions a day. "Any number of contractions done will probably improve bladder control," she added.

Whatever the number, it is important to make each contraction as strong as possible and to hold it for three seconds, then relax for three seconds. It is also important to identify the muscle in order to contract it correctly. This can be done most easily by stopping and starting the flow of urine. When contracted, the muscle will produce a sensation of pulling up or drawing together the external genitalia. Since it can be done any time and in any position, it would not be too difficult to get in even as many as Dr. Kegel's three hundred in the course of a day. One should notice a marked improvement within two or three months.

A woman told us recently that she had had trouble with stress incontinence because of a tilted uterus which caused some pressure. Her doctor told her that exercise did not do much good. He advised, "Let's get your uterus out. You're thirty-three and don't want more kids anyway." She ended her story by saying, "That was six years ago. Exercise did help me gain better control in a few months. And I still have my uterus."

How is a hysterectomy performed?

The surgery may be performed in one of two ways—with an abdominal incision or through the vagina. The technique used depends upon the patient's condition and the surgeon's preference. One of the gynecologists we interviewed explained that originally the vaginal procedure was used only in the case of a prolapsed uterus. But now many of his colleagues do vaginal hysterectomies routinely and do them very competently. However, this doctor said he still preferred to make an abdominal incision because with that procedure he could see more clearly the condition of the ovaries and surrounding organs.

Because the vaginal surgery does not involve an abdominal incision, the recovery period should be shorter. Some surgeons point out, however, that postoperative complications are more likely to develop. In Joann Rodgers' article, she cites doctors at Yale University who say that fifty percent more fevers and forty percent more urinary tract problems develop with vaginal hysterectomies.

The advantages and disadvantages of each procedure should certainly be discussed thoroughly with one's surgeon. And we urge any woman who has doubts about the decision to ask for another surgeon's opinion.

Whichever procedure is used, when a surgeon removes the uterus and cervix, the end of the vagina is folded up and sewn back like a cuff. When this heals properly, there should be no difficulties with intercourse or in any other way. Occasionally scar tissue will form at that point, but it seldom causes trouble.

The doctor who described this procedure for us emphasized that women who have had hysterectomies should still have a Pap smear taken at least once a year because changes could develop in the vagina or on that cuff.

When should ovaries be removed?

Frequently the question arises whether a woman approaching the age of menopause should have her ovaries removed at the time of a hysterectomy.

If there is any suspicion of a malignant condition, of course there would be no question. But what if the ovaries are healthy? Their production of estrogen is tapering off, it is true, but there is evidence that in some women the ovaries may continue to secrete low levels of estrogen until as late as age sixty. There is also some evidence that the ovaries continue to produce androgens, the male hormones, indefinitely. Not only are these androgens important in themselves to the body's hormonal balance, but there is evidence that some may also be converted into an estrogen through a process still not well understood.

On the other hand, many surgeons believe that the ovaries can be a source of trouble later, so removing them during a hysterectomy is a sensible precaution.

At an international symposium on menopause held in Atlanta, Georgia, in 1973, doctors from three different countries (Belgium, Canada, and the United States), were given the hypothetical case of a forty-five-year-old female having a hysterectomy for a nonmalignant uterine disease, and were asked whether they would remove the ovaries. They agreed that if the ovaries appeared normal, if there were evidence that they were still producing estrogen, and if there were no suspicion of a malignancy, the ovaries should be conserved.

Also if there were some reason why the patient should not be given additional hormones, the ovaries should be retained. One of the panelists also admitted that the surgical procedure might influence the decision. Sometimes it is difficult to remove ovaries during a vaginal hysterectomy, if their position is high in the abdomen.

Statistics concerning the incidence of ovarian malignancies and other types of disease also influenced the doctors' opinions. One study indicates that one or two patients out of one hundred might develop benign cysts, and another study, that three patients in ten thousand might develop ovarian cancer. One of the panelists asked if it would make sense to subject women to unnecessary prophylactic removal of ovaries when the risks of disease are comparatively low.

The panelists did agree to two exceptions, however. If a patient has a strong family history of ovarian cancer involving a mother or sisters, or if the ovaries appear to be involved in pelvic inflammatory disease, they should be removed, even though they appear to be normal.

The discussion concluded with a statement familiar in the study of menopause: "Continued work is necessary" to answer the many questions still remaining about endocrinal changes which occur in the menopausal process.

How should a woman decide what to do?

The decision about whether a patient should have a hysterectomy is not only up to her and her doctor. Most hospitals have strict regulations governing the performance of such operations. The surgeon must demonstrate that there is an indisputable reason for the surgery. So the day of the casual, "hysterectomy-by-choice," advocated by the doctor quoted at the beginning of this chapter, seems to be far off.

But even keeping all these questions and qualifications in mind, we think women who are advised by their doctors to have hysterectomies should not be frightened away from the decision. Although there are always risks in any surgery, today the hysterectomy is, in most cases, a safe operation when performed by a competent surgeon. And it can make life more pleasant for the woman who has been plagued with heavy and unpredictable bleeding, recurrent infections, or abdominal pain.

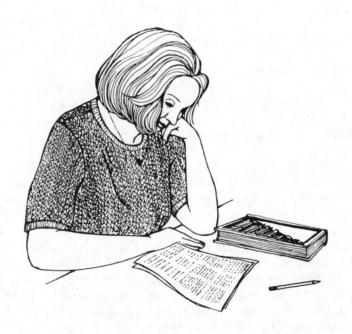

7

What Happens to Sexuality?

All this "openness" about sex
in magazines, books, and television —
it sounds like Show & Tell in the bedroom — makes me
uncomfortable. I begin to feel as if I'm
expected to turn into a regular sexpot.
At my age? I'm not sure I have the energy —

From a discussion at the YWCA

Of course, at any age a woman's physical and mental states affect her sexual experiences. But during the menopausal years she may run into special difficulties. At the same time, many middle-aged women feel reluctant to talk much about this aspects of their lives.

We've received comments ranging from this one in a letter —

"All the magazines tell you how you're supposed to enjoy sex more than ever after menopause, but I'm completely turned off. My poor husband thinks I don't like him any more and I love him dearly."

— to this remark made during one of our discussions —

"Don't tell me menopause turns you off sexually. I'm back in school to brush up on my bookkeeping training. And, I hate to admit this, but some of those young men look really good to me. It makes me realize how unexcited my husband has become about our sex life. Without too much effort, I bet I could get something going here."

83

The three of us who worked on this section disagreed about just how to handle the subject of sexuality and menopause. I wondered whether the subject needed special consideration, since it is so widely discussed everywhere. But Irma and Julie, who have had a good deal of experience talking with women—both in groups and individually, argued that it required a separate section because they had heard so many questions about how menopause affects a woman's sex life.

We decided an interesting way to describe how our ideas developed would be to include the following transcription of one of our editorial discussions.

Irma: The point I always emphasize when I talk to groups is that physical problems may develop during menopause, but they can be corrected. The most troublesome one—the narrowing and drying of the vagina—can be treated with an estrogen cream or ointment applied locally, or with estrogen pills taken orally. Or, leaving estrogen out of it, Masters and Johnson say that if a woman continues having intercourse regularly, she may not develop that symptom at all.

Julie: A woman might not want to come right out and discuss a problem like painful intercourse caused by a dry vagina, yet she should kow that it's not unusual and not difficult to treat.

Jane: I can see that that kind of information is important. It could forestall all kinds of problems. It's these sex specialists who are forever spouting advice on television and in books and magazines that get me down. Have a problem? You name it—they have the answers. Let's not come on like experts.

Irma: Certainly not. We're not professionals, anyway. But sometimes I think we're as "expert" as they are. I've read most of the books they've written. And more than that, I've listened to other women talk. ·

Julie: Some of those books are helpful, though. We will include a list of them for any women who want to read some more.

Irma: And in criticizing experts who sound too glib, we should not dismiss all sex therapy. A woman might get important help from a competent therapist. She should make sure to check credentials and methods, though. There are some real phonies around, I understand. We can suggest some books that will help there, too. Books that explain exactly how therapy is conducted. If it's a couple having problems, for example, the consultations usually include both a male and female therapist, not to act as surrogates, but to make communication easier. Or if a woman is nonorgasmic, she could talk with a female therapist who would understand her feelings and could teach her techniques to overcome the problem.

Julie: One positive thing we should emphasize is that after menopause, most women do actually seem relieved that the threat of pregnancy has come to an end.

Irma: Yes, but lets be sure to caution our readers that they should continue some kind of dependable birth control method for one year after their last menstrual period.

Jane: For sure. Let's enjoy grandchildren, if we're lucky. But spare us those menopause babies.

Irma: Another thing. It is generally agreed now that risks of high blood pressure, clots, edema, and heart attacks, which are associated with birth control pills, increase as you get older. So another method of contraception is desirable — spermicidal foam, a diaphragm, or condoms.

Jane: Some women are afraid of losing interest in sex altogether. What shall we say to them?

Irma: Some do notice a diminishing interest in sex, in "libido," to use Freud's term. Some doctors believe estrogen might help there, too.

Jane: But we don't want to get in the position of advocating hormone treatments. Especially when we've just cautioned against the use of birth control pills.

Julie: You're right. But, of course, the pill has much higher levels of estrogen than most women take for menopause. We should give the information we have and urge women to make up their own minds. And consult their doctors, too.

Jane: But many doctors aren't very comfortable about talking to middle-aged women, especially about sex. So by providing this information, we should make it easier for women to ask for help without embarrassment.

Irma: To get back to "libido," let's face it, if a woman has never cared much for sex anyway, she's not likely to be turned on after menopause. I guess there are still some women around who feel like saying, "Thank goodness, I can forget all that now. I've done my duty."

Jane: Maybe. But I would think that attitude would have been more typical of our mothers' times.

Irma: Just think how our mothers influenced us. It's really surprising that most middle-aged women, when given the chance, seem to enjoy a healthy, active sex life.

Julie: There's another thing we should include in this discussion—how men are affected by age, too. And how a man's attitude may influence his wife.

Jane: But let's make clear that men don't go through menopause. It irritates me to see magazine articles and books, there was even a television special recently, about "male menopause."

Irma: Especially since women haven't had a TV special yet about honest-to-God menopause. If men have never menstruated, how can they stop?

Julie: But men do face problems with aging too, both physical and emotional. And too often a woman will tend to take all the blame herself if things go wrong, especially with sexual relations.

Jane: And go out and buy another jar of Eterna night cream, if she can afford it.

Irma: Or the man will dump his wrinkly wife to take on a smooth young one.

Jane: I hope I live long enough to see some of these middle-aged swingers start to creak, while they struggle to keep up with their young women.

Julie: But seriously, it's hard for men to age too in our society. We put so much emphasis on virility and strength.

Irma: Yes, I can imagine it's pretty scary for a man when his ability to respond sexually — to achieve an erection or ejaculation — slows down or even fails him altogether.

Julie: That's when some men think the excitement of a younger partner will revive them, I suppose.

Irma: While, really, if a man and his wife understood that responses just slow down a bit as they get older, they would probably work things out quite easily.

Julie: It's not just physical, either. Imagine how an ambitious man must feel when a younger man — or woman, these days — gets the promotion he had counted on.

Jane: Or when he has to admit that he never will be a champion, at work or play.

Irma: Or when his sons and daughters tell him he's out of it these days.

Jane: I suppose the sex experts I've been complaining about might intimidate men as much as women.

Julie: In a way, it's harder for them because they don't seem to have the chance to talk about their anxieties the way women do with friends over coffee or in rap groups.

Jane: I keep hearing that men don't get chances to visit like that, but I wonder whether men would confide in each other, even if they had the opportunity.

Irma: Probably not. Even with friends, men seem to have to maintain that façade of control and strength. Can you imagine a man admitting to his friends that he was feeling a bit wobbly about his masculinity?

Julie: No, but just think how much it would help a man who is fearful about his future to know that others are having similar problems.

Irma: Now wait a minute. So far we've talked about women with husbands. Let's not forget all those women who aren't married.

Jane: But just because a woman's unmarried, and middle-aged, doesn't mean she can't have a sex life. Remember the woman in one of our groups who said she had not been sexually awakened until she was divorced at fifty? She and her husband had been raised to be very inhibited about their bodies. And though they had had children and been happy as parents, they had never been able to relax and enjoy each other physically. She said she had gone through a kind of late adolescent period after her divorce with lots of sexual experimentation. And she considered it a very positive force in her life.

Julie: But not all women have such chances, especially during middle age. As we just said, most older men seem to look for younger women. And our society still seems to frown upon women dating younger men.

Irma: And with women living longer, there are fewer men available as the years go by.

Jane: We have to remember too, that lots of women choose to live on their own. And seem perfectly well satisfied with celibate lives. Remember the woman who wrote to us not long ago who said she was proud not to have built her life around sex. For fifteen years since her divorce she has lived without a man. And has enjoyed every minute of it, she said.

Julie: And others have partners of the same sex. Even though young women these days seem open and accepting about lesbianism, most older women are still uncomfortable about the whole question of homosexuality. It seems only reasonable, though, that there are just as many lesbians among older women, but they are quiet about their life styles. So that's another choice for some women.

Irma: Another sexual option that most middle-aged women would find even harder to talk about is masturbation. Masters and Johnson call it "self pleasuring," certainly a better expression. They believe attitudes even toward that long-standing taboo are relaxing as more older women discover it to be an acceptable substitute for sex with a partner.

Julie: And some young women advocate the experience of masturbation as a way of heightening other kinds of sexual excitement.

Jane: But ideas like that run so directly opposite to all the standards of behavior we have grown up with.

Irma: I agree. The most important thing we can do is to

assure women that aging in general and menopause in particular need not alter a lovely sex life. That's one pleasure that can go on indefinitely — one way or another — for as long as one chooses. As that woman wrote in her letter last week, "After twenty-six years of marriage, sex is as great as ever. It's the best invention our Lord ever created."

The conversation which follows is an excerpt from a tape recording which reveals one reason middle-aged women often feel inhibited about discussing their sexuality. A group of old friends reminisced about their "education" concerning sex. Each woman had heard about it from her mother, but the manner of the telling varied dramatically. And that made all the difference.

Anne: Frankly, even at my fifty-odd years (and believe me, they do feel "odd" sometimes), I'm uncomfortable talking about sex. It's so important how your introduction to this whole sexuality thing is handled. Any information I was given was in my darkened bedroom with my mother obviously uncomfortable, stumbling through these guarded — and garbled — explanations. And mine was such a reserved family besides. My parents never showed any affection for each other. It took me years before I could relate warmly to anybody — especially men.

Doris: When my mother told me, she stressed how difficult it had been for her because her mother had not told her about the facts of life. And, as I remember, she never really got around to explaining it very well either. Anyway, I'm like you, Anne, I remember it as being a gray, depressing kind of experience.

Edith: My mother didn't tell me much either. So I was determined to do a better job with my daughter because I was enlightened. And I thought I did do a really thorough job. But years later she said to me, "Mother, you never really told me anything about sex."

Wilma: I think these explanations have to be personal and very concrete. My mother did a good job. She started with the emotional aspects, how much she loved my dad. I remember she told me while she was ironing. She said I would go through changes as I grew up. And she used the right labels for everything too. Then she asked me how often I thought they had intercourse and I said, "Well, you have five children and two of them are twins—four times." And she said, "Oh no, Honey, you've got it wrong. We have it many times because that's one way we show our love for each other.

Doris: Your mother deserved some kind of prize for enlightenment.

Wilma: Yes, the only stigma she put on it was you only do this after you're married.

Doris: I dreaded telling my daughter about menstruation because what I wanted to tell her was how exciting it is to be a woman. But at that point I didn't feel so good about it myself. I'd run into so many roadblocks of discrimination in my work and had just come out of an unhappy marriage. But I did find it easy to be warm and loving, and I did feel a special bond with her that day.

Anne: Well, that was probably the very best thing you could have done, then.

Wilma: It's funny how hard it is to judge sometimes what your children are really understanding from these explanations. When my grandson came home from school the other day, apparently having had some experience with a film or lecture, he said, "Grandma, did you know that there's this terrible thing that happens to girls on the first of every month?"

Edith: Yeah, especially if they're bookkeepers.

Anne: Looking back now, I wonder how I could have been so dumb about sex. I remember reading a play once about a woman who had had an illegitimate baby. I even remember the title, *Coquette*, with pictures of Helen Hayes. So I decided that you had a baby when you spent a whole night in a hotel room with a man. But I couldn't see how that would work, either. It wasn't until I got into high school and took biology that I understood.

Doris: I was like that too. I remember looking up *rape* in the dictionary once. And that was no help. It said, "Carnal knowledge without the person's consent." Then I looked up *carnal* and that said, "of the body." Well, I already knew that!

Edith: All my mother told me was, "Pretty soon you'll be menstruating." That was the first time I'd heard the word. "And you'll bleed a little from here," she said. Well, I'd always thought my mother had some pretty irrational ideas anyway. And I just considered that another one. I remember thinking, Maybe *you* do." When it finally did happen, the only difference it made in my life was that I couldn't walk to the library at night any more. No explanation. It was just forbidden, and I'd been doing that every night for years. I finally decided it had something to do with Des Moines because that's where we were living at the time.

Anne: All I can say is at least things are better these days. I took my four-year-old granddaughter to the store the other day. And as we were driving along in the car, she said, "Can you guess what I'm doing, Gamma? I'm jiggling my vagina." I was proud of myself. Without cracking a smile, I just answered, "That's nice, dear."

––––––––––––––––––

At the end of this discussion, even those who had spoken impatiently about their mothers' fumbling efforts agreed that the poor women could not have done differently when one considered how miserably they, too, had been prepared for sex and marriage.

To get a professional opinion about our treatment of sexuality and menopause, we sent the material to Professor Elaine Smith, an instructor in family education at North Seattle Community College, with an extensive background in sexual counselling. We conclude the chapter with excerpts from her letter of evaluation because she not only comments on our discussions, but adds constructive ideas of her own.

September 30, 1976

Dear Friends,

I like the chapter, especially the conversation about the women learning "facts of life," and its upbeat conclusion.

There has been so much "Hooray for sex" in books and magazines that I'm sure we're all getting a bit weary of the over-sell. On the other hand, you don't want to suggest that middle-aged sex has lost all its zing—even if that is the stereotype.

About the alternatives to heterosexual activity. I agree with you that masturbation is a very difficult subject for women who were raised to believe that it is an infantile practice that one outgrows at about age six. But even so, I find that "most" middle-aged women do, or at least have, masturbated, even though it does run counter to standards they were raised with. They just feel guilty about it. Perhaps if masturbation were treated in your book as an acceptable activity, there would be, not more masturbation, but less guilt. Certainly a positive contribution to women's feelings about themselves.

As for lesbianism, I find same-sex physical behavior more difficult for middle-aged women to deal with than masturbation. Or even to conceptualize. Many say, "What do women *do* together?" Without criticizing lesbianism, I would like to emphasize the importance of close, intimate relationships among women that include affection, respect, and trust, but are not genitally oriented. Not just from the practical point of view that many older women will be left without men, but because all humans need that kind of warmth to feel alive. But I'm afraid too many of us are reluctant to get close to other women because it might be "misunderstood."

Finally, I would like to give special support to those enduring relationships—usually long-standing marriages—in which affection remains strong, even though actual genital intercourse takes place infrequently. I suspect lots of couples, married for thirty-five or forty years, live this way quite happily. Besides the general slow-down in sexual performance that develops naturally with aging, lots of people don't realize that often medications, especially those for arthritis, hypertension, and other conditions frequently found in the middle years, can also reduce libido. Yet all this popular literature keeps throwing at them standards they find impossible to maintain. "If you don't have intercourse once or twice a week, you're going to shrivel up and fade away," can be pretty threatening advice to couples who enjoy intercourse once every month or so and maybe twice a week on vacation.

Many of these couples have evolved patterns of sexual sharing with one another that are exciting and satisfying to them. Rather than exclusive dependence upon genital coitus, they frequently incorporate massage, mutual touching and fondling, and oral sexual behavior in their physical relationship.

I hope these ideas will help.

Good Luck,

Elaine Smith
Family Life Education
North Seattle Community College
Seattle, Washington

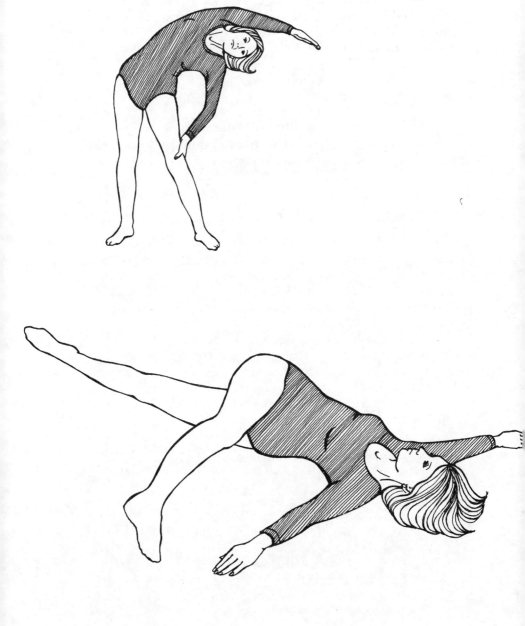

8

What About Life's Other Changes?

Not long ago in one of our discussion groups, a woman said, "I really appreciate that song that goes,
      Changing, always changing,
      Tomorrow I wonder who I'll be?
It describes my life exactly these days. It's scary, but in a way kind of exciting."

Someone else replied. "That makes me uncomfortable — the idea that I could change so much I don't know who I'll be. I want to believe there is a permanent center in me that won't ever change, no matter what."

These two reactions to change — its excitement and its threat — express the conflicting responses most people probably experience at one time or another as their circumstances and attitudes shift about throughout the years. But a middle-aged woman, especially during menopause, must feel the impact of change more than most. So much can happen at once. Not only does her body undergo changes, but often other patterns in her life alter drastically too.

A woman wrote to us recently, "It seems as if everything in my world is coming apart at the seams at once. My youngest son has turned into the typical teen-age terror, my daughter wants to leave home and move in with her boyfriend, my husband missed his big promotion, and now my mother's coming to live with us. All this when I'm bugged by menopause and feel weepy about coping with anything. And my doctor tells me I wouldn't be troubled by menopause symptoms — if only I'd get my mind off myself!"

So far, we have emphasized the physical aspects of menopause because we believe they are usually the cause of emotional tensions which may develop, ranging from occasional irritability to more persistent depression. Too often women are made to feel inadequate by those who insist that their problems are "in their minds." During a time of turmoil, how much does it help a woman to tell her, as one medical pamphlet does, that common complaints like insomnia, irritability depression, and fatigue "are the result of self-pity, frustration, or brooding about growing older. . . . you should take stock in yourself."

Such "common complaints" more likely result from shifting hormone levels, made worse by any number of the emotionally stressful situations our correspondent described. A friend said recently, "I'm just plain tired of facing one family upheaval after another."

Of course, physical and emotional tensions feed upon each other; sometimes it is hard to tell which comes first. The social scientists who identify external pressures as the principal cause of the symptoms women suffer during menopause are probably partly correct. Some of their studies also provide broader perspectives on contemporary American life.

A few anthropologists, for example, have tried to examine other cultures to see how women experience menopause in nonwestern societies. Unfortunately, they have found little information, partly because anthropologists (who have been predominantly male in the past) have not investigated menopause, and partly because their subjects have been reluctant to talk about such a private matter.

In one of her early books, *Male and Female*, Margaret Mead did state, "Where reproductivity has been regarded as somewhat impure and ceremonially disqualifying—as in Bali— the post-menopausal woman and the virgin girl work together at ceremonies from which women of child-bearing age are debarred. Where modesty of speech and action is enjoined on women, such behavior may be no longer asked from the older woman, who may use obscene language as freely as or more freely than any man."

Another anthropologist, Ruby Weitzer Morris, found that women in a small East Indian community which she studied (the Chhattisgarhi), were allowed to dance publicly after menopause. Some of the old women even chewed tobacco and took snuff or opium.

Pauline Bart, a sociologist studying depression among middle-aged women, reached the general conclusion, after reviewing several cross-cultural studies (including Aleuts, Navajo, Samoans, and peasants in Burma, India, and the Philippines), that, "It appears that in each culture there is a favored stage in the life cycle of women. For instance, if a woman has high status when she is young, her powers and prestige can be expected to decline as she matures, and vice versa."

So while the specific examples cited from other cultures may seem quaint from a twentieth-century American perspective, they might well represent a new freedom gained by these women as they grow older, a freedom which has wider significance in their achievement of higher status in society. They also make one wish there were some special privileges to be gained in our society by growing older. A widely-applauded rite of menopause would certainly be welcome.

Studies like these, which show how an individual's reactions and perceptions of herself are influenced by her cultural traditions, are of value in understanding ourselves, but they do not express the emotional tensions individual women experience as they find their life patterns changing. To describe some of these more immediate feelings, we want to let some women speak for themselves.

For several months *Women in Midstream* tape-recorded conversations with different groups of middle-aged women about the kinds of problems they had encountered in recent years. The project grew out of our frustrations when we first started organizing discussion groups. A number of women had indicated on our questionnaires that they would like to discuss their experiences with others, so we arranged for some meetings. In many cases women would come once, talk candidly about their feelings and worries, promise to return—and never show up again.

At first these "no shows" discouraged us, then we decided that some women needed one opportunity to relieve pentup emotions and that was all. They just did not want to reveal more of themselves. But so many of these conversations were filled with valuable insights that we wished others could hear them too. So we hit upon the idea of recording them. There was nothing scientific about our procedure, though we tried to choose topics which represent typical changes menopausal women face with their families, their work, their life styles. We gathered three or four willing participants together, threw out a subject, turned on the tape recorder, and let it happen.

Here are excerpts from five of those tapes, brief sections of much longer conversations—some lasted an hour or two. We have transcribed segments which reveal women honestly expressing their emotions and talking about ways to cope with a variety of situations. While none of these women relate their problems specifically to menopause, the changing patterns they describe typify those that many women face at that time.

The first conversation reflects differences in attitudes which might almost be described as "cross-culturtal"; at least the women involved see society adopting standards which seem alien enough to represent another culture entirely. One of them starts the conversation by expressing her resentment toward "those women's libbers" who seem to be telling her she should "expand her limited existence":

Beth says angrily, "I'm fed up with all of them telling me to change my whole way of life. It seems as if they've changed the rules in the middle of a game that I have played very well up to now. Why, when my babies were born in the 1950s, I was some kind of heroine—three kids and a clean house—that's what everybody said I should do! Now they tell me I should find 'fulfillment' by going to work. Well, I'm at home working like a dog."

She was talking with four friends who meet together regularly for lunch. They had watched a television interview with Gloria Steinem and were wondering whether she had anything to say to them—a group of middle-aged housewives. Three of the others agreed with Beth.

Phyllis: I'm with you, Beth. I resent these people telling me I should go out and get a job. My daughter's the big feminist now, and she even criticizes me for doing volunteer work. Here I've thought all these years I was doing some good, especially in my work with the Children's Society. Now she tells me I'm exploited because I'm not being paid for my time. I like to feel I can give something of myself, without expecting anything in return. My daughter says that's because I've been programmed to be a "nurturer." Well, I say, "Why not?"

Fran: But it's not just liberated women who put us down. I have to tell you what happened to me recently. I was on the board of a big community organization, and they decided to include in their annual report a short biography of each board member. There were some important names—a surgeon and banker and a couple of profs. When the chairman phoned to ask me about my occupation, I said, "housewife." His answer was, "We don't want to put *that* down. Haven't you ever done anything you were paid for?"

Anne: You should have hung up on him. The creep. At parties people are forever asking me what I do. I'm still trying to think of a good answer. If I say, "housewife," then they ask what my husband does. Next time it happens, I think I'll just say, "I'm a free-lance person."

Ellen, the fifth member of the group, had heard her friends out with growing impatience. Now she broke in. "Let's get back to Gloria Steinem for a minute. What she is talking about is the freedom to choose what we want to do. And I'm all for that. I worked for ten years—it was a crummy, routine job, I admit—but now that our kids are grown, I can choose to stay home. And that life suits me perfectly. I can work when I want and play when I want. And, by God, I dare anybody to tell me that's not a neat way to live. Besides, it takes a lot more self-discipline to live like that than when some boss is telling you what to do every minute. I say, we've got to respect ourselves before anybody else will respect us."

But according to another group whose conversation we recorded, a housewife's life is not always as idyllic as Ellen suggested. These women had been active at one time or another in the University of Washington YWCA and supported many of the changes advocated by feminists which break down rigid sex-role behavior. They had tried to incorporate some of them into their own lives, but had discovered that others did not always share their enthusiasm. Old habits die hard.

Kay started out by telling about her husband's reactions to sharing the housework:

Kay: I've been having quite a time lately. All these years I told myself that it was my job to do the housework because my husband was off working. Well, now he's out of a job. And this man, that I've been saying all these years is a feminist, that he understands women's feelings, is sitting around not doing a damn thing. I know he's going through hell with a personal crisis. So I don't want to light into him yet, but as soon as he gets his feet on the ground, things are going to have to change. I'm going to try to find a job to get us by—if I can at my age. I find myself doing those dishes and wanting to scream and just throw them against the wall.

Alice: Maybe you should try it sometime. Say it's those menopause blues.

Kay: Then again, I'm feeling sorry for him. But at least now I'm able to ask without any guilt feelings, "Would you do the dishes?" But I do have to ask. That bothers me.

Alice: For a lot of us there are stages we go through. And that's one of them—always asking, "Would you?" I remember Saturdays when my husband always watched television, seemingly endlessly. And he would say "Is there any coffee? And I would think, "Why is it that I'm in here working and am supposed to leave what I'm doing to make him coffee?" I decided he could make his own. That was a great moment.

Gwen: A stage I went through was to thank my husband for everything he did in the way of housework. Then I decided I didn't have to do that. That was a giant step for me.

Janice: It's funny. I seem to react just the opposite from the rest of you about my husband sharing the housework. I find myself resenting it. He tends to move in and take over. I feel sort of engulfed, especially since the kids left home. I guess it's his idea of togetherness, but I could do with less of that. I've worked out my own schedule over the years. And I don't need his help now. I feel like I'm being replaced.

Alice: I guess a lot of women run into that when their husbands retire and hang around the house all the time.

Janice: God help me. I should live so long. You know, I think a lot of men still believe the little woman can't quite cope. The other night my husband started to give me directions on how to go to the airport so I could pick up my mother. Imagine. I've lived here all my life. And he's going to draw me a map.

Gwen: To be honest, sometimes I really enjoy playing the part of the helpless female. Sitting back letting a man take over. It's so convenient. When the car won't start or the toilet overflows, I say to myself, "That's man's work."

Kay: But, Gwen, that's a trap. It makes you so dependent. And then you can be such a victim.

Alice: You mean when your husband throws you over for a younger woman?

Kay: Or collapses with a heart attack. I don't mean to sound ghoulish, but statistics show most of us will be on our own at the end of our lives.

Gwen: I know, we really have to be able to look after ourselves. In the long run, it makes for a better marriage anyway.

The three women in the next conversation no longer worried about how to make their marriages work out — they were all divorced. In comparing notes on how they had learned to live on their own, they agreed that, though some of their experiences had been bitter ones, they had come through as stronger people in the end.

Ruth has been divorced for more than twelve years, Avis for eighteen months, and Peggy's second marriage ended three years ago.

Peggy: When my second husband left, I was so demoralized at first I couldn't even get myself together to pay the bills. And I had worked and looked after household expenses for years.

Ruth: I got into trouble with charge accounts. During my marriage that had always been my pay-off for being a good wife — buying things on credit. In six months I was so far in debt it took me months to get my head above water after I found a job.

Avis: I haven't had much trouble with credit because I had a job before the divorce and had established credit in my own name. But a friend of mine was simply devastated when, after her divorce, the department store where she had traded for twenty-five years wrote requesting that she turn in her credit card — her charge account had automatically been cancelled.

Peggy: Well, I suppose the store had no way of knowing whether she could pay her bills.

Avis: Surely they could have given her the chance to prove she would pay before cutting her off like that. I told her I hoped she would never set foot in that place again — even if they do have the greatest white sales in town.

Ruth: The hardest thing for me after the divorce was simply accepting my singleness. For months I still kind of went along in the same kind of life I'd led when I was married. My friends were always kind about including me in their plans. Then I began to feel like a fifth wheel and decided to live in a different way, more on my own. I felt funny about going to singles dances, but I began to meet new and interesting people when I started doing other things. The best of all has been the photography class I'm taking at the community college.

Avis: People had warned me about that "fifth-wheel feeling" too, Ruth, when I decided to get a divorce. And I said, "Not to me, it won't happen." But I began to feel husbands didn't especially like to have me around because it might give their wives ideas. And wives were afraid I might give their husbands ideas. In fact, one of my former husband's best friends did offer me his — um — companionship. Maybe at fifty-three I should have been flattered, but I'm afraid he made me mad instead.

Ruth: I had a friend who used to call me up occasionally and say, "My husband's going to be out tonight. Why don't you come over?"

Peggy: Yet I just couldn't have made it without some of my friends. They were so patient about letting me groan and gripe about everything during those first bleak days. I'll never be able to repay them for how much they helped by just listening.

Avis: And you can't get that from your children either. When I try to get some advice from my daughter, she says,

"Mother, you have to start making your own decisions some day, you know." The first time she said it I was crushed. But now I guess she's right.

Ruth: That loneliness is still hard for me. And I've been divorced a long time. I didn't want it either. He just left. The classic case of the younger woman. Ever since, I've wanted to get married again.

Peggy: Really? I've been married and divorced twice, and now I find myself wondering, "Why do people ever get married in the first place?" Of course, I wouldn't have missed having children for anything. I've learned more from watching them grow up than they ever learned from me. And they're developing into independent young women, thank God. Sure, I get lonely, but what's wrong with being lonely sometimes, anyway?

Ruth: Yes, there is something to be said for learning to enjoy being by yourself sometimes. It does give you a great feeling of independence and strength.

Peggy: And happiness. It's wonderful to find out that you're a pretty neat person to be with, after all.

The fourth group of women talked about their jobs. They are old friends who meet for potluck suppers every three or for months. When they first started getting together, they were all at home with young children, but over the years they had found jobs, ranging in status from part-time secretary to full-time librarian. On this evening some of them looked back over their experiences and wondered whether they had made the right choices. Rehashing past mistakes is usually futile, but sometimes it helps a person see herself more clearly.

Their conversation also reflects the statistics which show that although the rate of women over forty-five joining this country's work force has increased dramatically since 1950, according to the United States Department of Labor, "mature" women, especially those who had dropped out of the labor market for several years to raise families, encounter difficult obstacles in returning. Among the disadvantages are "rusty or outmoded skills, no recent experience, and lack of job

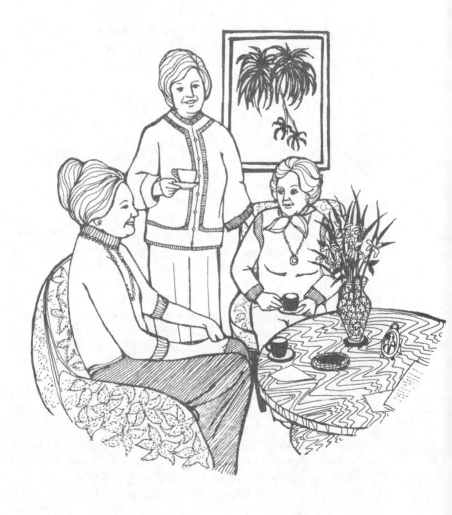

contacts." So those women who decide to get out and work, either because they must support themselves or because they seek new challenges, too often receive a disheartening reception.

Marie, who does part-time secretarial work, confirmed this kind of experience, saying, "I think back over the choices I've made, if it had to do with my work or my family, I always decided in favor of what seemed best for my family. Once I was offered an office-manager's job, but it was several hundred miles away and the family didn't want to move. Looking back, it's not a matter of what I should have done. I just lived that way. But I do feel resentful sometimes because I think I have as much on the ball as people who have careers for which they are well paid. They get recognition. And I would love work that I could feel involved in—which I certainly don't have now."

Doris was glad she had made a different decision about her family, but now is angry about suffering twin barbs of discrimination—against her age and her sex.

"I guess I was lucky," she said, "because I had opportunities. But besides, I had some kind of drive that made me feel like I had to have something else. I went back to school to train for social work when our youngest was in the third grade. And it was the best thing that could have happened to our family. It gave the rest of them the feeling that they had some responsibility for what went on. But I'm also fifty-three years old. I'm the only professional in our office, and I'm the lowest paid and I'm the lowest grade level. I live in a world that's almost totally masculine. I travel on planes where I'm often the only woman, and most of the men think I'm somebody's secretary. And at my age, I'm too late to ever catch up."

"You ought to work in the library," Helen broke in. "There it's almost totally staffed by women, and yet the higher echelon is practically all male. It seems as if almost any profession run by women is bossed by men."

"Do you know why I think that is?" Doris asked. "I think most women feel it should be that way. Even in my gut of guts I really accept the fact that men should run things."

"Well, I don't feel that way. I'm mad most of the time. I've worked in that library for nine years and suddenly, without a word of praise or a word of criticism, I'm on probation. They've given me a new job category, so I'm on trial for six months. I sure hope I make it because I'm getting old—I'm fifty-seven—and where else can I get a job? One of the other women at work said, 'If that happened to me, I'd hire a lawyer and I'd say, "What in hell do you think you're doing?"' But I'd be afraid I'd never work again. That's one of the ways they get rid of people. Besides, I would get the reputation of being a bitch. Let's face it. It's not to a woman's advantage to be aggressive. Even other women don't like it. So the men just smirk because they're impregnable—you should pardon the expression."

Now Jessie, the fourth member of the group, spoke up, "I guess the years have mellowed me. Where I work I wouldn't take the next job up for anything. They even offered it to me and I turned them down. It's too much of a hassle. I don't have that kind of energy any more. Besides I'm happy with what I'm doing. And I can get along with what I make now. Sometimes I feel like a fink when the young women in the office urge me to go higher. But I don't want that for myself. I will support them every time, though, in their ambitions. I'll do anything I can to help them get ahead."

All the women we recorded did not feel as positive as Jessie about young women's ambitions and desires for independence. The participants in this concluding conversation admitted to serious reservations about their daughters'—and sons'—life styles.

In her study of other cultures, Pauline Bart also found that women who live in societies where they are assured an established, important kinship role, like a mother-in-law or grandmother, adjust more easily to aging. One of the women in this conversation does express her concern about missing out as a grandmother, but the others seem more anxious about the apparent instability of their children's lives, as compared to the family patterns they have known.

These women had not met before we got them together at our office, but as often happens among strangers, they found this made it easy to talk about some of their private worries.

Kitty: The kinds of changes that I see tearing up families these days are the new ideas about sex without marriage. I agonized over it for months when my daughter announced she was moving in with her boyfriend. It was worse for her father. He's even more old fashioned than I am, I guess.

Alma: And besides, it was "his little girl" who was doing it. I have to admit to still having the old double standard, too. I wasn't nearly as upset about our son living with a girl as I was when our daughter tried it with her boyfriend.

Kitty: This is terribly old fashioned too. But I still think a woman invests more of herself in that kind of relationship than a man. It's partly biological, the feeling of privacy and specialness about her body that I just don't think men feel. And because of that, there's more emotional commitment for her too.

Alma: Do you think you might be interpreting the situation from your point of view, though? I don't believe very many young women would feel like that today.

Kitty: All I know is my daughter was much more distraught about it when she and her—what?—"live-in friend" broke up than he was. Of course, apparently he already had another girl lined up to look after him.

Alma: That's what gets me. I think a lot of these girls are being played for suckers. They're doing all the wifely things, with nothing to show for it in the way of property settlements when they do split up.

Meg: Who has property these days? I don't have a daughter, just two sons. And the thing that drives me nuts about them is they still don't know what they want to do. And they're both in their twenties. They're still talking like the flower children of the '60s. They just look at me blankly when I try to tell them things are different today. They're all grown up and life is real, life is earnest. And what in hell are they planning to do?

Kitty: Are you still supporting them?

Meg: No, one drives a cab till he gets enough money to live awhile, then quits and travels and writes poetry till he runs out of cash. The other one is on a run-down farm with some friends "living off the land," he says. I say he'd never make it if it weren't for food stamps.

Kitty: They're probably too gentle for our competitive times. Maybe theirs is a sensible response to times like ours when there don't seem to be enough jobs to go around anyway.

Alma: Here I go again sounding awfully old-hat. But wouldn't the job situation improve if some of these young women would stay home and have babies instead of demanding their rights to careers? Besides, I'm dying to be a grandmother.

Meg: Gosh, Alma, I can't believe that's the solution to talk about these days. You just can't tell ambitious young women to go back into the kitchen and nursery like we did.

Alma: I suppose not. But it makes me mad to hear my daughter say she won't have children because of overpopulation. I know things can't go back to where they were. That we're living in times of great change. But I still wish I could count on a big family dinner on Thanksgiving, with babies around instead of guitars and dogs.

Though these conversations may have raised as many questions as they answered, we hope they show how women can help each other out by sharing their feelings. Hearing about others' experiences can put one's own life into perspective, perhaps even cut one's problems down to size.

The conversations also show, we think, that those who can adjust to changing life-patterns become stronger for the experience. They may wonder "who they'll be tomorrow," but it will be a new person of their own choice.

9
What Can Women Do For Themselves?

I think doctors are playing
guessing games about menopause.
Women had better figure out things they
can do for themselves.
From a letter to
Women in Midstream

From the beginning of this project we planned to conclude with positive and specific ideas about Things Women Can Do For Themselves.

Everybody agreed that recommendations about exercise should come first. We decided to turn mainly to friends and correspondents for this information, describing activities which they themselves enjoy.

There was no dispute either about advocating a wholesome diet. However, this turned out to be more difficult. Of all the controversies we have encountered in studying menopause, those about nutrition are among the fiercest. We are not qualified to take sides. But not many doctors are either. It's a wonder the American public hasn't suffered a collective nervous breakdown, with all the conflicting information fed to them about what they should and should not eat. We have received advice ranging from the doctor who advocates the Hunza diet (named for the long-lived people of West Pakistan), to the friend who believes in vitamin therapy, with some vegetarian advocates in between.

We decided our most useful course would be to include basic information about weight recommendations, nutrient and calorie requirements, and the food sources for those requirements. We have also listed some of the more popular publications which deal with specialized approaches to nutrition and dieting, for those who want to investigate the subject further.

Our recommendations about organizing discussion groups grew out of our experiences at the YWCA and those of some other women in the community. The interview with an experienced group leader is intended to provide guidance both in conducting groups and in choosing leaders.

The advice about evaluating health care has also developed from our experiences with people asking about choosing doctors and interpreting medical information published in newspapers and magazines.

The final section, made up of answers from a number of different women to our question, "How do you feel about the age you are now?" supplies, we believe, honest and positive statements about how it feels to grow older in a society like ours, hung up on the advantages of staying young.

So in answer to the question, "What can women do for themselves?" we respond: Exercise, Eat Well, Talk Together, Evaluate Your Health Care, and Appreciate Your Age.

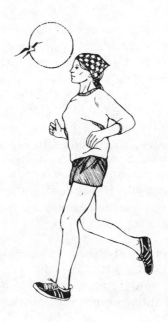

EXERCISE

Some women respond to our emphasis on exercise by saying, "Good grief, I'm so busy now, there aren't enough hours in the day. And you tell me I should exercise? That's what I do all day now." But everybody needs recreational exercise too.

We can quote any number of testimonials from individuals about the exhilaration they enjoy in their special activities. Among them are:

Bicycling

"Once I caught on to shifting gears, I found I could cycle as well as ever. It's not just that it's good exercise, but I feel so free gliding along. I remember what it felt like to be ten years old again."

Tennis

"My friends and I must look pretty clumsy, galumphing around the tennis court. But it's done wonders for me. The absolute concentration it requires to coordinate my head, hands, and feet in order to hit the ball shuts off all my other worries. When we finish, I have to stop and think, 'Now what else was on my mind:' "

Skiing

"Last winter I took up cross-country skiing. I was never much good at regular skiing, but this kind is great. Not much trick to staying up on them, and the scenery is breath-taking."

Dancing

"I've joined a class that combines exercise and dance movements. At first it was just an excuse to wear leotards—which has been one of my secret desires for years. But then I made an exciting discovery—there is still strength and grace in my body. Muscles I've neglected for years are being stretched and limbered. And, surprisingly, without pain or strain."

Swimming

"I still think swimming does it all. I go to the pool at our downtown YWCA at least once a week. You can use practically every muscle in your body, yet with little effort or strain. You can work at it hard or paddle around the edges like I do—I'm no Esther Williams, you understand. You can even do calisthenics in the water, if you want to."

Jumping Rope

"My doctor suggested I needed some vigorous exercise, enough to make my heart beat faster and my breath come quicker. She says just walking is for people over eighty-five. But jogging makes my feet ache. So I got my daughter's old jump rope. I'm just skipping along at a leisurely pace now, but pretty soon I'll work up to "cross overs" and "double time.""

Walking

"My favorite exercise is still walking. But not just strolling along. I keep a brisk pace, three to four miles an hour. And I consciously stride out as far as I can, so my muscles really stretch. It's most fun if I go with a friend so we can visit too, but now I don't even mind going alone. I try to walk an hour a day, then I can throw away those sleeping pills."

Even all the doctors we interviewed were unanimous in emphasizing the importance of exercise, especially for postmenopausal women. Besides generally improving the body's functions, exercise helps to maintain healthy bone structure. As a person ages, the bones naturally tend to thin out and become less dense. Since women have less bone mass to begin with, this process affects them more than males. If the condition becomes severe and the bones very brittle, it is called osteoporosis. Until recently medical researchers theorized that the loss of estrogen after menopause was the major cause of the condition. But that theory has come into question. Now most authorities believe that regular exercise and an adequate diet are the most important factors in preventing this potentially troublesome condition.

Also as a person ages, the muscles tend to lose their elasticity and the joints stiffen up. Regular exercise will combat these tendencies too, in keeping the body supple. Maintaining firm abdominal muscles is especially important because they help to hold the internal organs in place and to prevent their sagging into a prolapse. Also, weak abdominal muscles are a major cause of back aches.

With these benefits in mind, one can see that regular toning-up calisthenics are as important as recreational exercise. Here are some routines which friends have recommended as being helpful in counteracting physical weaknesses middle-aged women may develop. Of course, each person should check her physical condition, especially blood pressure, with a doctor before undertaking any of these.

And another word of caution passed on by a friend, "If you're going to advocate exercise, please warn your readers not to try to keep up with those television experts. They're in fantastic shape and make everything look so easy, you're tempted to overdo. I tied my back in knots, doing sit-ups with Jack La Lanne."

Flexibility

"I'm pretty stiff when I get up in the morning, especially when the weather is cool, so I have trouble creaking through calisthenics. Now I've worked out a routine of stretching my muscles in bed, before I get up. First, I lie on my back and breathe deeply several times, moving my abdomen up and down. Then I stretch my right leg down toward the foot of the bed and my left arm up toward the head, then relax. Repeat with the left leg and right arm and relax. Then stretch out both arms and legs at the same time and relax.

"Next I raise my head up till my chin touches my chest. Repeat this a few times.

"After this, my blood has started to circulate some, so I throw back the covers, bend one leg, grasp the knee with both hands, and pull the leg up toward my chest. Repeat this with the other leg. Repeat, alternating legs, a few times.

"These routines don't exercise all my muscles by any means, but when I do get up, I'm limber enough to do some calisthenics without too much trouble." —Janine

"These two are my favorites for stretching stiff legs and back. I like to do them first thing in the morning. But start out slowly and never overdo.

"To the count of eight stand straight, hands behind your neck, elbows out.

"To the count of four, bend over until you feel the first pull in your back. Rest there for four counts. Bend over further, with legs still straight and hands behind neck, as far as it is comfortable. Hold for four counts. Drop arms, bend knees, relax neck, arms, and rest of the body. (Fingers may touch the floor.) Hold for four counts. Keeping buttocks pulled in, gradually straighten legs as you rise, reaching hands straight over the head and stretching. Repeat three or four times. You will find that you can bend over much further the fourth time than the first.

"I call the second one *Swinging.*

"Stand straight, hands over head. Bend over in squat, dropping hands. Keeping body bent, straighten legs and swing arms back. Then bend knees and swing arms forward. Rise to standing position with arms over head. Repeat as rapidly as you can several times."　　　　　　—Eileen

"Recently I took some yoga lessons put on by the park department. The class is finished now, but I still do some stretching routines every day. Yoga is great because the emphasis is never to strain yourself, yet you can stretch all over. The positions have exotic names, but many of them are quite simple. Here's one I like especially because it limbers up your spine.

"Sit on the floor with the knees drawn up to the chin.

"Clasp hands underneath the knees.

"Lean forward, rounding the back. Press the forehead against the knees.

"Roll back onto the spine, hugging the thighs tightly. Keep the back hunched and the legs together.

"Use the recoil momentum to return to the starting position.

"Rock backwards and forwards several times. Breathe evenly throughout."　　　　　　—Maribeth

Muscle Tone

"Here is an exercise for the abdominal muscles which I learned from a physical therapist.

"Lie on your back on the floor with knees bent, heels apart and close to the buttocks, and toes turned in. Grasp your thighs under the knees and pull your legs up to your chest. Open your legs to the sides and slowly lower them, pushing against the resistance of your hands. Slide your feet back to the starting position. Breathe easily all the time. Repeat the exercise three or four times, always going slowly."　　　—Virginia

"A routine that is in most of the yoga books I've read is supposed to be good for "massaging the internal organs,' but I do it for exercising the abdominal muscles. It is recommended that it be done five to ten times, three times a day, and *only before eating*. And it should not be done during menstruation or pregnancy. You should be careful not to overdo this one. It seems simple, but it can make the muscles sore.

"Stand erect, legs comfortably apart. Lean forward and place the palms of the hands on the thighs, just above the knees.

"Exhale fully through the nose and mouth. When all the air has been expelled, draw the relaxed abdomen back and up towards the spine, creating a hollow in the abdomen.

"Hold the retraction for one second, then relax the abdomen and breathe normally again for a few seconds before performing the next retraction." —Eloise

"I wonder whether anybody else is concerned about accumulating fat on the hips like I am. I've decided the best exercise for this is to sit on the floor with legs straight out in front and arms at the sides, and roll back and forth, pressing weight on one side then the other. Or you can do a fanny walk by pushing yourself from one side to the other with your hands and moving forward then back across the floor." —Helena

"Several years ago I learned some dance exercises from a women's magazine. I've always liked them because you're supposed to do them to slow waltz music. Since that's not so easy to find on the radio these days, I just hum 'The Blue Danube' to myself while I do them — it keeps the pace slow and easy. Here's one that's supposed to trim the waist.

"To a slow count of three, step to the right with right foot, and draw the left foot behind it. (Turn out the toes of your left foot to keep your balance.) At the same time, raise your arms overhead, and sway to the right. Repeat movement with the left foot, swaying to the left. Start with five times on each side; gradually increase to ten times on each side." —Sheila

Relaxation

Relaxation routines are not exactly exercises, but they may help to relieve two of the most common complaints women suffer during menopause — nervous tension and insonmia. Two women told us that they have even lowered their blood pressure by conscientiously doing relaxation routines twice a day. We do not have any firm evidence that such techniques have helped with the relief of hot flushes, but it seems likely that they should.

We have included several books which describe useful techniques for relaxation in the Suggested Readings list.

Since insomnia is another common complaint of menopause, we pass along here a routine which one of our correspondents "guarantees" puts her to sleep every time:

"I've worked out a routine which always puts me back to sleep when I wake up—usually around that hideous witching hour of three in the morning. It's partly psychological because now I don't get worried; I just say to myself, 'O.K. time to empty out my head and go back to sleep.'

"First, I lie on my back and concentrate on breathing deeply, thinking about how my abdominal muscles rise and fall.

"Next, starting with my toes, I tighten all my muscles one after another—toes, legs, hips and abdomen, waist, chest, and at the same time, hands and arms, finally neck, and even face.

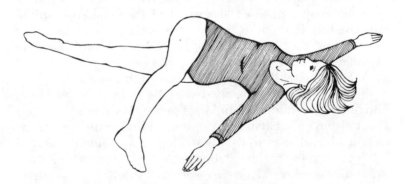

I lie for just a second or two with all the muscles tense, then suddenly relax all over. I breathe deeply again several times then repeat the tensing and relaxing. Repeat the whole routine two or three times.

Then, and this is what I find the most important part, lie in the most comfortable position and concentrate on emptying the mind. The best way to do this is to pick out a word and repeat it over and over again. I say 'nothing,' because I find the sound and rhythm of it relaxing.

"Not only do I go back to sleep, but it is such a restful sleep, I always wake up refreshed."   —Eloise

EAT WELL

For most middle-aged people, eating well means eating less. As one grows older, the basal metabolism changes so that the body requires fewer calories to maintain the same weight. Since overweight can contribute to serious complicatons like high blood pressure, heart trouble, and even diabetes, the individual will probably have to control her diet more carefully than before.

One woman told us recently she had found that cutting down on her meat consumption and substituting fish and chicken helped her control her weight.

Another said she had given up her evening cocktails when she discovered how many calories there are in liquor. "Now I settle for a glass of wine before dinner and make sure it's dry because sweet wines are loaded with calories too," she added.

Someone else wrote that just eating less of everything in her regular diet kept her weight in line. "But I've always eaten lots of fruit and vegetables," she explained. "This way I don't have to hassle with dieting and calorie counting, which takes the joy out of eating for me."

The woman with the "sweet tooth" probably has the toughest problem. One told us recently that she begins to crave sweets so desperately that she is trying the "Saturday Night Special" method. Once on the weekend she allows herself a truly horrendous treat like apple pie à la mode or a chocolate sundae, then eliminates desserts for the rest of the week. Another said she allows herself one tablespoon of ice cream or sherbet after dinner to satisfy that life-long dessert habit.

Here is a table from a government publication, *Heights and Weights of Adults in the United States*, which lists recommended weights for given heights. Tables like these are based upon desirable weights at ages twenty-five to thirty because a person should try to maintain that weight for the rest of her life. Of course, with statistics like these, general body build has to be considered too. That is why this table lists three weights — low, median, and high. Those with small bones would be classified as *low*, while large-boned people would fall into the *high* category. If a person's weight is within ten percent (over or under) of that recommended for her height, her weight is about what it should be.

Weights for Women
(without clothing)

Height in Inches (without shoes)	Low (Pounds)	Median (Pounds)	High (Pounds)
60	100	109	118
61	104	112	121
62	107	115	125
63	110	118	128
64	113	122	132
65	116	125	135
66	120	129	139
67	123	132	142
68	126	136	146
69	130	140	151
70	133	144	156
71	137	148	161
72	141	152	166

A reminder about calories. Though nutritionists talk about "low and high calorie foods," humans do not really eat calories. When carbohydrates, fats, and proteins are used by the body, heat is produced. That heat production is measured in units called calories. Foods vary in the number produced:

- Carbohydrates produce 4 calories per gram,
- Fats produce 9 calories per gram,
- Proteins produce 4 calories per gram.

If the amount of energy needed by the body is less than that supplied by the diet, the extra energy will be stored as fat, and the person will gain weight.

This chart from the U.S. Department of Agriculture shows how calorie requirements decrease with age.

Women Total Calories			
Weight (in pounds)	25 years	45 years	65 years
88	1750	1650	1400
99	1900	1800	1500
110	2050	1950	1600
121	2200	2050	1750
128	2300	2200	1800
132	2350	2250	1850
143	2500	2350	2000
154	2600	2450	2050
165	2750	2600	2150

Another element to be considered in controlling weight is one's weight will influence the number of calories burned. For example, during a one-hour walk a 110-pound woman may burn up 100 calories, while a 190-pound man on the same walk may burn 173 calories. Also walking up a 10% grade burns twice as many calories as walking on the level. Or walking on sand uses up more calories than on a sidewalk. Weather also makes a difference. In colder weather a person burns more calories to keep warm.

Type of Activity	Calories per Hour
Sedentary, such as: reading, writing, watching television or movies, sewing, playing cards, typing, and other activities done while sitting that require little or no arm movements.	80 to 100
Light, such as: preparing and cooking food, doing dishes, dusting, walking slowly, and other activities done while standing that require some arm movement.	100 to 160
Moderate, such as: making beds, laundering by machine, light gardening and carpentry, walking moderately fast, and other activities done while standing that require moderate arm movement.	170 to 240
Vigorous, such as: heavy scrubbing, stripping beds, walking fast, bowling, golfing, and heavy gardening.	250 to 350
Strenuous, such as: swimming, tennis, running, bicycling, dancing, skiing.	350 and more

A person must think about more than just maintaining a desirable weight, however. As one ages, a balanced diet is as important as ever. The simplest way to assure an adequate diet is to choose foods from the *Four Food Groups* each day: milk and cheese; meat, fish, and eggs; vegetables and fruits; bread and cereals.

Postmenopausal women should remember two other things about their diets. First, it is neessary to eat adequate amounts of calcium for the maintenance of bones. And remember the body also needs vitamin D to absorb that calcium. Dairy products are the richest source of calcium. These include: whole, skim, dry, or buttermilk; cottage cheese, yogurt, and hard cheeses—cream cheese and butter are not good sources. Some vegetables and seafood provide calcium too. Several women have told us that they take calcium pills, usually in the form of bone meal, but whether that is necessary is open to question.

The second aspect of diet which is often important to post-menopausal women is the limitation of sodium in their food. High levels of sodium may lead to excess water retention (edema) which is associated with high blood pressure. It is important to remember that salt is not the only source of sodium, though it is the principal one. Baking powder, baking soda, and monosodium glutamate are other common sources. Women who take diuretics to counteract edema should also be sure to keep adequate amounts of potassium in their diets because much of it may be eliminated with the excess fluid.

Among the many controversies about nutrition, one that appears high on the list is whether "natural" foods are more desirable than "processed" ones. Since valuable nutrients are lost in the refining of most foods, especially in grains like wheat and rice, it would seem sensible to choose unrefined products when possible. Many of these foods also provide the roughage which is essential to efficient elimination. Also, since consumers are hearing warnings from every side about the possible dangers of chemical food additives, it again seems only prudent to eat as many natural foods as possible.

This advice does not refer to the controversy about whether foods grown "organically" are superior to those produced with "chemical" fertilizers. In our opinion, the evidence is not in yet on that dispute.

We mention two other major nutritional controversies because they are so much in the news—not because we are about to take sides.

First, should one limit the amount of cholesterol in the diet? The body naturally manufactures cholesterol from fats and carbohydrates. It is a substance which is normally present in many tissues, but is especially important in brain and nervous tissue and in the liver. Cholesterol in the skin can be changed into active vitamin D by the ultraviolet light from the sun. So it is clear that it is a substance vital to the body. However, many doctors believe that when there is an excess supply of cholesterol in the blood, it, along with other fatty materials, is deposited in the linings of the arteries, thus narrowing the channel through which the blood flows. This arteriosclerosis is the most common cause of heart attacks and strokes.

According to this theory, with the restriction of foods high in cholesterol and the addition of polyunsaturated fats, a person may protect herself against these hazards. Foods to be restricted or eliminated include egg yolks; whole milk products; fatty meats, fish, or poultry; and solid shortenings. Corn, safflower, soy, and sesame seed oils are among the polyunsaturated oils which counteract the undesired effects of excess cholesterol. One should remember that some oil is essential in the diet.

Since this theory of the relationship between cholesterol and cardiovascular problems has been questioned by some authorities, we do not advocate such a diet. However, there are techniques for measuring a person's blood cholesterol levels, so we do advise anyone concerned about such a condition to consult a doctor before deciding what course to follow.

The second dietary controversy concerns vitamins and minerals. No authority disputes their importance; the question is whether one need take vitamin and mineral pills to supplement those obtained naturally from a balanced, well-prepared diet.

The "official" answer, the one most doctors provide, would be like that in the government bulletin, *Myths of Vitamins*: "Foods can and do supply most Americans with adequate nutrients, and consumers should not expect any major physical benefits from multivitamin pills, contrary to the myth."

On the other hand, many of the women who answered our questionnaire did take vitamin supplements regularly and believed they helped them maintain good health.

For further discussions on the subject, we refer any interested readers to the books on nutrition listed under the Suggested Readings for this chapter.

The following table, adapted from two government publications, lists the kinds and quantities of foods recommended for the "adult in health" and the nutrients supply by each. It is important to remember, in evaluating information like this, as one of the government books states, "present knowledge of nutritional needs is incomplete." As confused consumers, we can only hope that the researchers make rapid progress. In the meantime, it would be a sensible idea to eat as varied a selection of foods as possible to insure a balanced and wholesome diet.

122

Nutritive Value of a Basic Diet Pattern
For The Adult in Health

Food	Amount	Calories	Protein gram	Fat gram	Carbohydrate gram	Minerals Ca* gram	Fe** gram	A I.U.	Thiamine mg	Riboflavin mg	Niacin mg	Ascorbic Acid mg
Milk	2 cups	320	18	18	24	576	0.2	700	0.16	0.84	0.2	4
Meat Group:												
Egg	one	80	6	6	trace	27	1.1	590	0.05	0.15	trace	0
Meat, Fish, Poultry	4 ounces	240	33	10	0	17	3.6	35	0.32	0.26	7.4	0
Vegetable-Fruit Group:												
Leafy green or deep yellow	1/4 to 1/3 cup	15	1	trace	3	14	0.5	3590	0.03	0.04	0.3	14
Other vegetables	1/4 to 1/3 cup	20	1	trace	4	13	0.5	300	0.04	0.03	0.4	9
Potato	1 medium	80	2	trace	18	7	0.6	trace	0.11	0.04	1.4	20
Citrus fruit	1 serving	40	1	trace	10	18	0.2	150	0.07	0.02	0.3	42
Other fruit	1 serving	60	1	trace	16	12	0.5	600	0.04	0.04	0.4	9
Bread-Cereal Group:												
Wholegrain or enriched cereal	3/4 cup	105	3	trace	22	10	0.8	0	0.12	0.04	0.8	0
Wholegrain or enriched bread	3 slices	180	6	3	36	57	1.8	trace	0.18	0.15	1.8	trace
		1140	72	37	133	751	9.8	5965	1.12	1.16	13.0	98
Recommended Dietary Allowances												
For Women			55	—	—	800	18	5000	1.0	1.5	13	55
For Men			65	—	—	800	10	5000	1.4	1.7	18	60

*calcium
**iron

123

TALK TOGETHER

We have quoted from conversations and personal statements throughout the book to emphasize the value in talking with others about one's feelings and problems, whether they concern menopause specifically or life in general.

Of course, group participation isn't for everyone. One woman commented on her questionnaire, "Why would I want to blab to others about my health? That wouldn't help me or anybody else."

But many others have told us how much it has helped to discuss their problems. "The best that came from our group was the support we gave each other. Several men wanted to join to learn about menopause too," a woman wrote us recently.

Another told us how much she enjoyed being in a group with middle-aged women. "I enjoy young people. I work with them all day long, and I admire their energy. But it is so comfortable to visit with women my own age. I feel as if we have come out of the same world. They'll understand when I complain about my personal future shocks," she said.

Groups may take a variety of forms. The most successful one we have conducted at *Women in Midstream* continued for nine months. The group met one morning a week for two hours at the YWCA's offices. The size fluctuated from as many as ten to as few as four. A couple of women dropped out as other demands interfered, and a few new ones joined. Because the group was loosely structured the shifts in membership made little difference; in fact, the new arrivals often stimulated fresh ideas.

We were lucky to have a leader, Julie Campbell, who had considerable experience conducting discussions like these. Several of the women felt Julie was the key to the group's success.

"Her techniques were low-key, so we were scarcely aware of her direction," one of the women said. "But she set a pattern to begin with that was so helpful, we continued it throughout the year. We always started our discussion by having each person brag about something she had done for herself during the week. It was a simple device, but I found myself consciously doing something positive each week so I would have "a brag" to contribute. You wouldn't believe what a difference that made. We all developed more confidence in ourselves."

Another member said, "I wasn't aware of Julie's leadership until she was absent. Then I felt we wandered around too much in our talking. And one or two people tended to dominate the discussion."

"On the contrary," a third member argued, "I felt as if we came to know each other and to trust each other so much, we could function as a group without any special direction. The trust that grew among us was our great strength."

Since every participant in the group praised Julie's leadership, we asked her some more specific questions about her techniques, with the hope that her ideas might serve as a guide for others.

Interviewer: To begin with, Julie, you call yourself a *facilitator* rather than a *leader*. What's the difference?

Julie: I know it sounds a bit fancy, but there is an important difference between the terms. *Facilitator* means to me, "*We* the group will work through these questions or problems *together*," while *leader* implies, "I'll show the way and you follow." My goal is to encourage the group members to be independent—not to lean on me. In a way, when we start out I'm "one up" on everybody because I've had experience. But my aim is to equalize the power in the group.

Interviewer: How do you go about that?

Julie: For one thing I explain techniques as we go along. For example, when we first meet, I say that I want to begin each two-hour session by each one taking a turn at "bragging." The "bragger" tells the group about something she has done for herself, for her own satisfaction, during the past week. As an alternative (and this is often even harder), she can brag about at least one positive, unqualified aspect of her personality, like "I am intelligent" or "I have a wonderful imagination." I explain these are tools for building self-esteem, for discovering (or rediscovering) what pleases them, for learning to take time for themselves. In dealing with the difficulties in bragging, we might then discuss Transactional Analysis as a tool for diagnosing aspects of one's own personality. In discussing other ways of building self-esteem, we might explore the inherent creativity of one's own dreams. In talking about the frustrations women encounter in attempting to take time for themselves, we might discuss assertiveness training, anger exercises, or values clarification.

Interviewer: Then you encourage the women to read more about these different approaches too?

Julie: Yes, by all means, I always tell them about the books I've read or other places I've learned my techniques. I emphasize that these are different kinds of tools they can learn to use to work out problems, either in groups or on their own, outside the group situation. Besides, I emphasize that I am learning too. Women in each group constitute their own expertise. For example, in one group a nurse with a special interest in nutrition and massage became "the leader" when those subjects came up for discussion.

Interviewer: To go back to the beginning, how do you get a new group going?

Julie: One thing that's important in starting out is to set some ground rules.

Interviewer: Could you summarize them?

Julie: There are four basic rules we all agree to. First, confidentiality. Nothing said during our discussion will be repeated outside the group without that speaker's permission. I emphasize that we have to combat the stereotype of "gossiping women." And let me say, I've never known this to be a problem. Women take it very seriously. The second rule, listen to what others say without passing judgment (or pretending to sympathize, if you really don't). Third, don't give any feedback, as advice or otherwise, unless it's asked for. And fourth, don't put down the speaker—women already get plenty of that kind of discounting outside the group.

Interviewer: What if a person asks for advice? Do you give it then?

Julie: Yes, I usually encourage the others to give their ideas first. Eight heads are better than one when it comes to giving opinions. And, again, this is a way to emphasize that I'm not the "expert." Also it helps me to hear the others' suggestions first, then I can sum them up and maybe make some kind of general statement that everybody can relate to.

Interviewer: What would be an example of such a generalization?

Julie: Well, say one of the women tells about having been fired from her job. The others might not have had exactly that kind of experience, but if I make a generalization about the pain one suffers in facing any kind of rejection, everyone can think of such an incident in her life. The value in that kind of sharing is that it gives a broader perspective to one's own experience.

Interviewer: So if a response is asked for, you encourage everybody to participate.
Julie: Yes, with one exception. I do intervene if one person starts to put down another. I may even point this out explicitly. It's another way of teaching.

Interviewer: Several women have praised the technique of bragging which you use to start off.
Julie: That's another way women build confidence in themselves. It's a simple thing, but it works remarkably well. Middle-aged women, especially, have been conditioned to be self-effacing—to put others' needs ahead of their own. I really enjoy watching women grow from being wholly embarrassed by bragging to being practically addicted to it. It develops not only their self-esteem, but others' appreciation of their more positive attitudes about themselves. Setting up a loose structure like that also helps to get a group going each session.

Interviewer: One criticism we've often heard about group discussions, especially if there isn't a specific leader, is that one or two people tend to dominate. How can that be handled?
Julie: Structure can help a lot there. First, with the "brags," everybody gets a chance to talk. Then I will ask how many in the group have something they want to talk about and how much time they will need. Or we figure how much time is left, how many want to talk, and simply divide up the minutes. And I usually reserve some time for myself. My groups last two hours, so it usually leaves plenty of time for everybody. But with that agreement ahead of time, it's then possible to cut someone off by saying, "Time's up."

Interviewer: What if the group agrees to give most of a session to one person?
Julie: Well, that's O.K. Sometimes when a woman first comes into a group, she may have a problem so much on her mind that she can't even listen to others until she has had a chance to talk. Usually the group allows for that and is willing to

listen. However, women learn quickly to assert themselves and demand "equal" time.

Interviewer: What about someone at the other extreme who just listens?
Julie: Occasionally there are women like that. Of course, she has to contribute her brag, but if that's all she wants to say, that's all right too. It doesn't mean she hasn't gotten anything from the group. That's just where she is at that time.

Interviewer: How many women do you like to have in one group?
Julie: I work best with eight or nine, and not less than five. But that's an individual preference. Other leaders might like a different size.

Interviewer: What about having friends together in the same group?
Julie: I prefer that they don't know each other to begin with, certainly having relatives in the same group is not a good idea. My groups usually meet at one of the YWCA branches rather than in private homes, so the participants have the freedom to choose whether or not to continue their relationships outside the group. Most do, but it's helpful to have that option.

Interviewer: Are the groups set up for a definite number of weeks?
Julie: Usually they're set up for an eight-week series, but they can continue if the group wishes. Like the one here at *Midstream*, it went on for eight or nine months.

Interviewer: Isn't there a danger that a woman could become too dependent upon her group? That she wouldn't stand on her own?
Julie: But we're not striving to be completely independent — that's being a hermit. Even a strong person is dependent on others for some needs. No, what I hope is a person can come to recognize, accept, and respect her strengths as well as her weaknesses. That way she will gain more confidence in herself. Then she should be more able to function well in any situation. Or maybe she will want to join another type of group. I would expect a person to gain more confidence with each new group experience she has.

128

Interviewer: You have certainly shown how important leadership can be to a group. It's also clear why one of the women in the *Midstream* group described your guidance as "low key." You were apparently successful in making them independent because several felt they could function without you after a few months.

Julie: It's something like being a parent. As much as you might love it, you have to finally work yourself out of a job.

Interviewer: And like being a parent, I'm sure this all takes experience, but you have given us some valuable pointers, so women can try it themselves. Or, at least, you have provided some standards by which to judge others' techniques.

Though Julie's interview does show how a competent leader can keep a group running smoothly, some women we've heard from question the necessity for that kind of guidance. A friend who had been in a group outside the YWCA explained her attitude this way, "Women, especially middle-aged women, depend too much on authority figures. When our group first met, I stated this conviction very firmly and insisted that we could get along without a leader. Apparently two of the women didn't like the idea because they never came back. But those of us who continued did get along fine for the eight weeks we had agreed to meet. We learned to know each other well enough to talk quite frankly about what was bugging us. It sure helped me over some rough spots."

Another friend said her group had developed more of a structure as time went on. Originally they met together once a month for dinner and casual conversation. But some of them decided they needed more direction to their discussions. So now each time they decide upon a topic to discuss at the next session, and one of them agrees to be the moderator. "This way," she said, "each of us can read up on the subject, if we want to. We've talked about everything from social security to sex. And everybody gets a chance to add her two-bits worth. I've learned a lot."

Of course, groups do not have to be confined to personal discussions. During the summer of 1976 Irma Levine, one of the coordinators of *Women in Midstream*, wanted to emphasize our promotion of exercise, so she formed a *Walk and Talk Group*. It consisted of an eight-week series of short hikes

129

around the Seattle area. Each Tuesday the women met at a designated location, walked for two or three miles, then stopped for an hour to eat brown-bag lunches and talk about whatever was on their minds. The discussions were unplanned, but by the end of the series, the participants agreed that they had covered a number of important questions — besides improving their physical condition and endurance.

Another possibility, one which *Women in Midstream* may plan when the personnel and facilities are available, would be a combined information and discussion group. It would be limited to a four-week period, with the program specified ahead of time. Each two-hour meeting would be divided between a program presentation and discussion. Even this type of group would not require "experts" to conduct it. The women themselves could agree ahead of time to assume the responsibility for presenting the information at one of the meetings. A tentative program might follow the plan of this book: What Is Menopause? What About Hormone Therapy? What About Life's Other Changes? What Can Women Do For Themselves?

This information could also be presented in a one-day workshop, perhaps combining formal lectures with small group and panel discussions. This type of function requires more planning and publicity, but it can also accommodate larger numbers of participants. And some of them would probably want to organize subsequent groups of their own.

Some more informal groups we have heard about in our area meet for different purposes, but also offer their members the chance to talk over personal concerns. Like the friends who have been meeting together once a month for several years to discuss books — and incidentally their own problems. "We can hardly talk about Doris Lessing's novels or Elizabeth Janeway's essays without talking about ourselves too," one of them said. Or the women who for twenty years have celebrated each other's birthdays with potluck dinners. Or the group, described in a local newspaper, who go to concerts and ballets together because they live alone or their husbands are not interested.

The participants and the circumstances of each group will determine its structure. Some basic questions should be answered at the beginning: Will the group meet only for a specified number of weeks? Will the membership be limited in number? Will the topics for discussion be decided ahead of time? Does the group want a single leader or will it share the responsibility among its members?

For those who do not want the responsibility of establishing a group themselves, we suggest that they call a community organization like the YWCA or a church or community college and ask that such a group be established. In any community one may be sure that there are women who would welcome the chance to share their experiences with others.

EVALUATE HEALTH CARE

Choosing a Doctor

We frequently receive calls at *Women in Midstream*, asking us to recommend a doctor. This is a chancy business; one woman's root beer might be another's seltzer water. We will sometimes tell the caller about one or two doctors whom others have praised. But too often the word has already spread and such doctors no longer take new patients.

Sometimes it helps to ask the caller specifically about what she is seeking. If she is fed up with specialists and needs some general advice about her health, we suggest she call someone in family medicine. We also remind callers that many communities have more informal women's clinics. These are usually staffed by paramedics or trained lay people, and supervised by a doctor. A woman can be sure of finding a sympathetic ear at a place like that. On the other hand, if a woman with generalized menopausal complaints has consulted one gynecologist after another, we suggest she might see an endocrinologist for tests of her hormone balances. This kind of examination is usually expensive, however.

Another possible course of action is to check on the credentials of several doctors. This information will not give a clue to personality, but at least the prospective patient will learn something about the doctor's competency. County medical societies will provide the names of several doctors, specifying females, if asked, their educational backgrounds, and special training. Public libraries usually have the American Medical Association's Medical Directory, which also lists this type of information.

Though it is also helpful to know at which hospitals a given doctor has staff privileges, this information is a bit harder to come by. Probably a call directly to the doctor's office is the quickest way to find this out. That is also the time to ask about other details like office hours, fees, and the possibility of house calls.

Medical societies are under increasing pressure from consumer groups to provide all this information in readily-availble directories. But so far it is argued that keeping such information up to date would be too difficult. And furthermore, no one seems willing to finance such costly projects.

Asking Questions

Ours seems to be an era when the medical profession has become sensitive to patients' rights for a number of reasons. Not the least of these are consumers' demands for fuller information and doctors' anxieties about malpractice suits. These forces have coalesced to create a new atmosphere for openness. In Washington State, for example, under the impetus of a new law regulating health-care procedures, the state medical association has published a pamphlet which states, "When seeking medical advice or treatment, consider yourself as a participating member of the health care team. . . . As a participant, you should feel free to make suggestions, comments, or to ask questions about any aspect of medical treatment or diagnostic procedures prescribed."

Patients should take advantage of suggestions like these. As "a member of the health care team," tell the doctor about everything which is troublesome. Ask about anything which is puzzling. Some women tell us it helps to make a list of questions as a protection against the office jitters.

One of them explained, "I always used to make a list of questions to ask our pediatrician whenever I took the baby for a checkup because it was such a confusing ordeal. Now I do the same thing when I go to my doctor, so I won't be tempted to brush off complaints that begin to seem too trivial to mention in the hurried office atmosphere."

Another said once she had written her doctor a letter describing a special problem she was having, before she went in for an office visit. "My doctor is always pleasant enough, but her nurse is a witch," she explained. "She even intimidates me when I phone for an appointment, saying, 'What do you want to see the doctor about this time?' With the letter, I figured the doctor would hear all my complaints — and maybe have time to think about them before she saw me in person. It worked really well. I've never had to do it again. I think the nurse got the message."

If doctors want their patients to be "participants" in health care, they also have to talk in terms a lay-person understands. So ask for clarification of technical words. We have included a glossary of medical terms related to menopause which should also help in asking questions and interpreting answers. (pp. 159)

If a doctor prescribes a course of treatment, especially surgery, about which a patient has any doubts, she should certainly ask for another opinion. It is not a time to worry about "hurting the doctor's feelings." One can either ask the doctor for a referral or seek one out herself. In either case, the doctor should be willing to pass on any relevant medical information from patient records, including results of laboratory tests, X-rays, and physical examinations, to the consultant.

The legal question as to whether a patient has a right to her medical records has not been settled on a national level. State regulations on this question vary. However, the American Medical Association policy is that doctors are ethically obligated to summarize medical information for a patient, even if the records themselves are not turned over to that patient.

Checking Up

Another new tendency in medicine, probably to cut down on costs, is to discourage routine annual physical examinations as a part of preventative medical care. But this advice seems questionable to us. All women should have a Pap test at least once a year. And postmenopausal women, especially, should have a blood pressure check at that time.
We hope that by now all women do regular monthly breast examinations on themselves, but it is probably a wise precaution to have a doctor examine the breasts manually at the time of the Pap test and proceed with an X-ray if there is any question.

READING CRITICALLY

Women should have no trouble today keeping informed about medical developments. In fact, they are too often inundated with news, especially if it is frightening. If cancer or heart trouble is the subject, any report makes the headlines. While reading such news reports, here are some things to keep in mind:

Read beyond the headlines

Headlines may be inaccurate. The *Seattle Times* (November 24, 1975) headlined one story, "Menopause Weakens the Heart." In this case the reader had to go well past the first paragraph for an accurate interpretation of the information. It read, "When women go through menopause, they lose much of the protection against heart diseases they used to have through female hormones during the reproductive life, the American Heart Association reported."

Near the end of the story it is made clear that this is a highly speculative statement because the story concludes, "The investigators could not find an obvious explanation for the increase in heart disease after menopause." Dr. William B. Kannel, director of the study, is quoted as saying, "Evidence from animal and human studies suggest that estrogenic hormones may be partly responsible. . . . Still hormones don't seem to be the whole answer."

Headlines may be misleading. Another headline about the same reports, appearing in *The Wall Street Journal*, read, "Studies Hint at Link of Uterine Cancer, Menopause Therapy. They indicate Women Taking Synthetic Estrogens Have Greater Risk of the Disease." The reader might easily misinterpret this to mean that a distinction is being made between "natural" estrogen pills (like Premarin) and "synthetic" pills (like oral contraceptives), whereas the news story refers to the replacement of the body's own hormones by any type of estrogen pill.

Consider the Source

Generally, magazine stories give more detailed information than newspapers because they provide more space and time for reporting. Monthly magazines usually discuss a subject in greater detail than weekly news magazines, unless the latter do special reports on the subject.

In evaluating reports about medical findings, whether in magazines or in newspapers, it is important to consider the source of the information. Of course, a lay person cannot be expected to evaluate the standings of professional journals, but the following guidelines should be of help:

1. *Does the information result from the work of several doctors over a long period on large numbers of patients?*

The study reported in *The New England Journal of Medicine* (August 19, 1976) which raised questions about the relationship between estrogen therapy and breast cancer resulted from a joint project of the Harvard School of Public Health, the National Cancer Institute, and the University of Louisville School of Medicine. And it was based on studies of 1,891 women over a period of twelve years.

Contrast this to a study reported on in *Newsweek Magazine* (January 6, 1975) which suggested that estrogen therapy might be effective in treating chronic depression. Although it was described as "a strictly controlled experiment," four men (two psychologists, one endocrinologist, and one biochemist) from two institutions (the Worcester State Hospital and the Worcester Foundation for Experimental Biology) studied only thirty psychiatric patients, and their experiments were conducted over a three-month period. Half of the patients were given doses of estrogen and the other half placebos. So when they report that 80% of the estrogen patients improved, they are describing twelve persons.

This is not to suggest that these researchers are not following a promising path toward the treatment of depression, just to caution that at this time that is all it seems to be—a promise for the future. And while the study of the possible relationship between estrogen therapy and breast cancer must also be pursued over many years with thousands more women, those more extensive findings already reported, will carry great weight.

2. *Does the information come from a professional association?* Specialist groups like the American College of Obstetrics and Gynecology or health organizations like the American Cancer Society or the American Heart Association do not issue reports unless they have been studied and evaluated by committees of professionals.

3. *Does the information represent one doctor's opinion?* We have learned to be especially skeptical about columns of advice written by individual doctors.

First, they can be seriously oversimplified. In one such nationally syndicated column, "For Women only," by Dr.

Lindsay R. Curtis, he advised a forty-two-year-old woman to have a "complete" hysterectomy (he meant removal of uterus and ovaries), adding that "by supplying you with substitution estrogen, we can stave off the menopause indefinitely." Far from "staving off" menopause, such surgery can dump a woman into it by cutting off her natural estrogen supply. More correctly, he should have explained that hormone therapy could alleviate any symptoms brought on by the surgery.

Another weakness with such free medical advice is that it has to be so generalized that it cannot be applied safely to individual cases. An angry letter to another newspaper doctor illustrates this difficulty. It is addressed to Dr. Robert Mendelssohn. "Do you realize how many women hang on every word you write?" this correspondent writes. "Now they'll REALLY go into hot flashes and nerve spasms as they flush their Premarin down the toilet because of your 'advice.'" She goes on to explain that since her hysterectomy twelve years before, she has depended upon estrogen pills to get her through. This doctor's general attack on estrogen therapy would not apply to her, or possibly to hundreds of other readers, either.

So, as a final word of advice, even though a doctor may bristle at a patient who quotes medical findings from *Good Housekeeping* or *Family Circle* magazines, we still believe any woman who has questions about such information would be better off facing her doctor's momentary annoyance than stewing about questions in silence.

APPRECIATE YOUR AGE

We have tried to be honest at all times in this book—and positive whenever possible. But there is no denying that menopause does signal an end to one phase of a woman's life—her fertility. It is a reminder, too, that time is moving on. Our youth-ridden society does not make this rite of passage easy, either. If you cannot be young, women are told, for heaven's sake, act young, look young, think young, eat young.

Now it is time for women to ask—Why? "Young" is great while it lasts, but why hold on when the string runs out?

Doris Lessing, a British novelist, once said, "Growing old is really extraordinarily interesting." Most of the women we have talked with agree with her. Recently we asked a number of them, ranging in age from forty to sixty-eight, "How do you feel about the age you are now?" Their answers make clear that Lessing's "interesting" does not necessarily mean happy or easy: "challenging," would be nearer the truth. But most agreed that the loss of youth brings other gains.

Of course, the years bring some regrets. A friend answered our question this way:

"How do I feel about being sixty? I'd rather be fifty! There's really no difference between fifty-nine and sixty, both pleasant ages, exept the label. Once you move out of the fifties, you're no longer "middle-aged" How we used to hate that expression). You're . . . mature? old? a senior citizen? a gray panther?

"Goodbye, middle years! Maybe we can blame the sociologists. Age is a continuous variable, but they tend to divide ages into discrete categories: "under thirty," "over sixty," the better to analyze their data.

"One thing I've learned, though. It's better not to get attached to any age, because I'll soon be older."   —Hannah

Other confessions about the inconveniences which come with age included these:

"So many of my favorite store clerks have retired, leaving youngsters who don't understand what I want."   —Pearl

"I always seem to be at the 'Get Well Card' Rack." —Zoe

"I notice most authority figures in my life—doctor, minister, lawyer—are younger than I am now. I'm beginning to feel like *everybody's* grandma."   —Ingrid

The years bring some physical discomforts, too:

"I can't eat pizza, baked beans, or corn on the cob any more without my stomach growling in protest. Instead of the old refrain, 'Let's have another cup of coffee,/Let's have another piece of pie,' my theme song has become, "Let's have another cup of decaf,/Let's have another piece of toast (low in calories, high in roughage).' "   —Florence

"Pretty soon I'm going to be the little old lady in bare feet, not tennis shoes. I cannot face any more chic clerks in platform soles, who grimace when I ask for shoes with low heels, strong arches, and broad toes, so I can walk around town in comfort."   —Betty

But even women who feel out of it sometimes, usually manage to maintain a fighting spirit. One great difference between the first awkward age and second is that by the time the middle years have rolled around, most of us have developed an identity and sense of worth which cannot be shattered by fashion's whims.

This woman who wrote about shopping for clothes reflects that kind of strength:

"You ask me about my age at a bad time. I've just come in from a shopping trip. Looking for clothes these days makes cleaning the oven seem like a gala affair. What's happened to the 'dependable suit' of yesteryear? It's now in The Designer Salon and costs $350. And the 'dressy wool' that will go anywhere? It's nowhere.

"It's as if the garment industry has proclaimed that any woman who has outgrown Junior Miss should blow away or kiss her elbow and become seventeen again. If you can't wear 'now styles' from the Right-On Boutique, you've had it, madam.

"Well, I'll show them. I'm buying a sewing machine on time, and at long last fulfilling a life-time promise to myself by enrolling in the next sewing-made-easy class at the local community college.

"In the meantime I'll wear my old wool skirt with the waistband unhooked and the zipper half open. I'll cover it up with an old sloppy-joe cardigan, i.e., my 'classic wrap-around coat sweater.' These young squirts can't lay me away ahead of my time. I've got to wait around to see them spread out."
                                                    —Gladys (48 years old)

Even when the years have brought some bitterness, the same kind of strength shows through, as in this statement:

"I don't need men any more. Not only has the sex urge dropped back (I thought it never would), but I find that where I used to think of men as being straight-forward thinkers, I now see that they are not. They are frightened of their shadows, as well as of older women.

"I'm never sick. I have learned to control my arthritis with diet and exercise (no drugs with superbad side-effects), I don't catch cold. When I'm angry I pound on a pillow instead of getting sick. Last year I learned to tap dance and it is the perfect exercise for a loner.

"I'm more at society's mercy than I've ever been, but that also confers freedom. If society isn't going to be loyal to me, I have no obligation to be polite and loyal to it. I see less and less about society to admire since it gave me the old heave ho, and it is a refreshing feeling." —Esther (54 years old)

Strength was expressed by this woman, too, but in a more positive way:

"This year I wrote on my calendar, "Happy Birthday to me. Life begins at 67!" To be honest, I felt the same on my 50th.

"My young womanhood was a stark struggle with hard challenges: the economic depression, raising my family within a stormy marriage, losing my health and learning how to regain it.

"This year finds me physically fit and active, emotionally comfortable with my children, grandchildren, and people in general. My modest income permits me to keep a small house. I cut my own lawn and have a little garden, eat what I please and have become a vegetarian. Through the city's best annual rummage sales, I have clothes for every occasion.

"The ability to draw instantly upon previous experience whenever I am faced with an emergency is a resource which only years of living can give. I am beyond the shock stage. Either I can (a) cope with whatever faces me, or (b) it will kill me. So why worry?" —Judith

The freedom which comes with added years was the theme of several responses:

"Forty came in with a whimper. Heralded as a day for dying one's hair red, having a nose straightened, or buying a new wardrobe. I was amazed to find I had no inclination to indulge in any of these things. I like my age. I no longer have to pretend I would go skiing if I had the time. I'm not going skiing because it's too cold! I don't want to end up in a snow bank.

"At my age I know what I can do well. At last I'm at the age where I can decline the first grade's trip to the zoo in favor of writing, baking bread, or reading, without the mental gymnastics necessary for inventing an excuse. 'I'm sorry, I'd rather not,' I hear myself say, and then I delight in the sense of freedom."　　　　　　　　　　　　　　　　　　　—Lucille

"The week before my birthday, I knew the company computer was whirring away, gathering up all the vital statistics of my twenty years of work, figuring out all the benefits due me, and would stop at the number 65, when I would be automatically retired. Retired for what, I often wondered—old age? What would I do with all my time? I had heard that some women were bored, frustrated, or just plain nervous wrecks—they couldn't kick the work habit.

"I had been home free only two days, when I knew a new life and world had opened up for me. The hours of the day were my own to do as I pleased. Though I had enjoyed my work and my friends at the office, after the first week it seemed that I had not worked for twenty years at least.

"Old age? Well, it didn't come at 65, 66, 67, or 68, and I know I'll be too busy at 69 to be old."　　　　　　—Maude

"I've been thinking about what I like about my age—fifty-five my next birthday. I'm interested in things outside myself now. And this is a relief after all those years of worrying about 'What to wear,' and 'What would people think?' With this comes a relaxation of standards and a new tolerance toward others. A sort of 'What was all the fuss about?' attitude.

"Politically I am returned to the radicalism of my youth. That is a refreshing development. I guess it's all part of my not worrying about what other people might think. I certainly hope I don't live forever. Another twenty years will be plenty!"　　　　　　　　　　　　　　　　　　　　—Paula

One contributor expressed her determination to keep her mind alive:

"My bones may ache, but my mind's still clicking. On my fiftieth birthday—four years ago—I promised myself that every year I would try one new thing. That first year it was tennis (maybe that's why my bones ache). This year it has been growing strawberries. Next year I'm going to try photography. Who knows? I might even master chess. I'll never be an expert at any of them. But it's the trying that counts and keeps my brain alive."　　　　　　　　　　　　　　—Roberta

Perhaps the best gift the years can bring is the kind of serenity these two women have found in recognizing the continuity of life:

"I think I have come to terms with myself. My options may be lessening, but that also means I don't have to agonize over decisions any more. I also enjoy a sense of fulfillment, of reflecting on the life cycle of the earth which softens the impact of aging and death. Since they happen to every other living thing, why should they not also happen to me?"

—Teresa (52 years old)

"When I try to pin down how I feel about my age, I find myself puzzled because what's happening at the moment has so much to do with how I feel.

"For instance, one day my granddaughter says, 'Why are your hands wrinkled?' I look at my hands and see that indeed they are getting wrinkled. At that moment I'm hit with the realization of the inevitability of age, of the fact of my mortality and others' I care about. Then I feel sad.

"But on another day I sit at my dinner table with three generations of my family. My grandson looks up at me, and suddenly I see my son at that same age. My daughter tilts her head in a characteristic way, and I am reminded of my mother. At that moment I feel good about my age, glad to have come so far and to have been so lucky. Whatever the future holds, the past belongs to me."

—Rachel (62 years old)

Robert Browning's, "Grow old along with me, the best is yet to be," may overstate the case for the later years. But we hope these statements from some of our friends do ring true and will suggest some reasons for appreciating your age, wherever it falls in the progression of years.

We hope, too, that armed with information and encouragement from our book, every reader will look at herself with a new understanding of her own body and a new respect for her own possibilities.

HORMONE MEDICATIONS

We have included the following information about various brands of estrogen medications, compiled from the *Physicians' Desk Reference 1976*, because women often inquire about the particular pills they are taking. We do not mean to suggest that any one of these medications is better than another.

In one way, this kind of list is unsatisfactory because the drug companies specify the process through which the medications are produced—esterified, conjugated, or synthetic— but not all of them give the sources of the estrogenic substances used. *Equine* (as in Premarin and Femogen) indicates the source as pregnant mares' urine. *Synthetic* (as in Diethylstilbestrol, Estinyl, and Tace) indicates the source as chemically manufactured. The others do not specify their sources. At this time, the medical profession does not believe one type is any safer or more effective than another for treatment of menopausal symptoms.

The list does provide two important points of information for the general reader, however. First, the dosages, which in most cases are indicated by color. The list shows that synthetic estrogens are much stronger than the others, so the dosages are much smaller. This also makes the synthetics generally less expensive than the other estrogen medications.

The second important point of information is that some of the medications contain substances other than estrogens: Menrium and Milprem include tranquilizers, and Estratest and Os Cal Mone include the male hormone, testosterone. We point this out so that we may once again urge each patient to ask her doctor just what her prescribed medication contains and the reasons for her taking it.

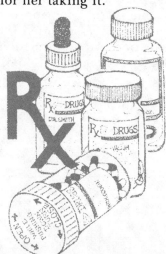

Medications With Hormones

Brand Name	Laboratory	Ingredients	Dosage *
Amnestrogen	Squibb	** esterified estrogens	0.625 brown 1.25 orange 2.50 purple
Estinyl	Schering	synthetic estrogen	0.02 beige 0.05 pink 0.5 peach
Estratab	Reid-Provident	esterified estrogens	0.625 yellow 1.25 orange 2.50 pink
Estratest	Reid-Provident	esterified estrogens and methyltestosterone (male hormone)	0.625 estr. 1.25 test. green 1.25 estr. 2.50 test. dark green
Evex	Syntex	esterified estrogens	0.625 peach 1.25 pink 2.50 yellow
Diethylstilbestrol	Lilly	synthetic estrogen	0.10 1646 J49 0.25 1647 J50 0.50 1648 J51 1.00 1649 J52 5.00 1685 J54
Femogen	Fellows	esterified equine estrogens	0.625 blue 1.25 turquoise 2.5 yellow
Hormonin #1	Carnick	estriol 0.135 estradiol 0.3 estrone 0.7	pink
Hormonin #2	Carnick	estriol 0.27 estradiol 0.6 estrone 1.4	green
Menest	Beecham	esterified estrogens	0.30 yellow 0.625 orange 1.25 green 2.50 pink
Menrium	Roche	Librium (tranquilizer) and esterified estrogens	5.0 Librium 0.2 estrogen blue 5.0 Librium 0.4 estrogen dark blue 10.0 Librium 0.4 estrogen purple
Milprem	Wallace	meprobamate (tranquilizer) and conjugated estrogens	200.0 mepr. 0.45 estr. lavendar 400.0 mpr. 0.45 estr. pink

(CONTINUED NEXT PAGE):

143

Brand Name	Laboratory	Ingredients	Dosage *
Ogen	Abbott	estrone sulfate	0.625 yellow 1.25 peach 2.50 blue 5.00 green
Premarin	Ayerst	conjugated equine estrogens	0.30 green 0.625 red-brown 1.25 yellow 2.50 purple
Os-cal-mone	Marion	calcium and methyltestosterone and estradiol	400 2.67 blue ***5.33
Sk-Estrogens	Smith Kline & French	esterified estrogens	0.30 white 0.625 yellow 1.25 orange 2.50 pink
Tace	Merrell-National	synthetic estrogen	12.0 green 25.0 two-tone-green 72.0 green and yellow

* All dosages are measured in milligrams unless otherwise noted.
** Esterified and conjugated are terms describing the chemical process used to produce the medication.
*** 5.33 micrograms

OUR YWCA QUESTIONNAIRE
(See next four pages)

Women in Midstream collected only enough money to have 250 of the more than 700 completed questionnaires analyzed by computer. Though the results are limited, some of them are of interest:

The respondents ranged in age from 28 to 73 years, with two-thirds of them between 45 and 55 years.

81% were married and living with their husbands. Most had children who were no longer living at home.

Half of the respondents described themselves "in the midst" of menopause and 16% "all through."

75% reported receiving hormone therapy, 45% had tranquilizers prescribed, and 11% were told no treatment was necessary. 15% received dietary supplements and psychiatric therapy was prescribed for 9%.

78% discussed their problems with female friends or relatives and half of them found this helpful. 69% discussed their problems with husbands or male friends and 46% found this helpful.

Menopause Study Group
Questionnaire

I.   PERSONAL INFORMATION

1. Age_____

2. Marital status: ☐ single ☐ married ☐ widowed ☐ divorced ☐ separated

3. Where do you live? with ☐ husband ☐ family ☐ friend
☐ alone ☐ retirement home ☐ other:_____

4. Do you work outside your home?_____
☐ as a paid worker   ☐ as an unpaid worker

II.   MEDICAL HISTORY (pertaining to reproductive organs)

1. Have you ever been pregnant?_____ How many times?_____
live births_____ still born _____ miscarriages _____ abortions _____

2. List your age for each of these pregnancies_____

3. At what age did you begin menstruating?_____

4. In the past, have your periods been ☐ regular? or ☐ irregular?

5. Do you now menstruate? ☐ regularly (every month) ☐ fairly regularly
☐ occasionally (2 to 4 times a year) ☐ frequently and irregularly (more than
once a month) ☐ not at all (over one year since last period)

6. Do you think that you are presently ☐ all through with menopause
☐ in the midst ☐ just beginning ☐ no signs

7. Is or was your menopause experience ☐ easy ☐ moderately easy ☐ difficult
☐ moderately difficult

8. Have you had your tubes tied (tubal ligation)? _____ At what age?_____

9. Have you had a hysterectomy?_____ At what age?_____
   (A) What was the primary reason for the hysterectomy? ☐ sterilization
   ☐ medical (tumor, cancer, excessive bleeding, etc.)
   (B) Did the hysterectomy bring on menopause?_____

10. Have you had any other types of pelvic surgery? (specify):_____

11. Have you had any breast surgery? ☐ for cysts or benign tumors ☐ cancer
☐ other:_____ At what age(s)?_____

12. How often do you have a Pap smear?_____When was the last time?_____

13. Do you know how to do a self-examination for breast lumps?_____

14. Anything which may be pertinent that you would care to add:

146

III. MENOPAUSE SYMPTOMS

The following are things that sometimes trouble older women and that may be associated with menopause (although they may also affect men and younger women). Please check any that have troubled you in the past or that currently trouble you. Put a $\underline{d}$ after problems for which you have seen a doctor.

- ☐ hot flashes
- ☐ muscle spasms
- ☐ profuse sweating
- ☐ tension headaches
- ☐ digestive disorders
- ☐ depression
- ☐ crying spells
- ☐ nervousness
- ☐ apprehension
- ☐ frequent urination
- ☐ unusual fears
- ☐ urinary incontinence (loss of control)
- ☐ abnormal taste
- ☐ osteoporosis (porous or brittle bones)
- ☐ burning sensation in mouth
- ☐ irritability

- ☐ constipation
- ☐ sudden back pains
- ☐ increased sexual desire
- ☐ decreased sexual desire
- ☐ weight gain (more than ten pounds)
- ☐ weight loss (more than ten pounds)
- ☐ insomnia (can't sleep)
- ☐ loss of memory
- ☐ age spots
- ☐ excessive fatigue
- ☐ dry or irritated vagina
- ☐ vaginal hemorrhage
- ☐ heart palpitation
- ☐ unable to control emotions
- ☐ allergic reactions
- ☐ other:

IV. DIAGNOSIS AND TREATMENT

Medical opinion differs considerably on treatment for menopausal symptoms. If you have sought treatment from a doctor for any symptoms you have had, please indicate the treatment(s) she/he suggested.

1.
- ☐ no treatment necessary
- ☐ barbituates (phenobarbitol)
- ☐ amphetamines (pep pills, diet pills)
- ☐ nutritional supplements (diet, vitamins):

- ☐ psychiatric therapy
- ☐ tranquillizers (nerve pills, sleeping pills)
- ☐ hormone therapy (estrogen or combination)
- ☐ specify other:

_____   _____

_____   _____

_____   _____

2. Were you satisfied with the doctor's attitude?_____

3. Was she/he helpful?_____

4. How many doctors did you go to with your problem(s)? _____

5. Have you consulted anyone other than doctors about these problems?

   ☐ clergyman   ☐ mental health worker   ☐ women's clinic worker

   ☐ social worker   ☐ specify other: _____

6. Was she/he helpful?_____

7. Have you discussed these problems with female friends or relatives?_____

8. Were they helpful?_____

9. Have you discussed these problems with husband, male friends or relatives?_____

10. Were they helpful?

V. NUTRITION AND GENERAL HEALTH

Many authorities believe that menopause difficulties can be reduced by careful attention to nutrition.

1. Do you think you are eating a balanced diet?   ☐ yes   ☐ no   ☐ not sure

2. Are you taking any form of vitamin/mineral supplement?   ☐ vitamin A

   ☐ D   ☐ C   ☐ E   ☐ B-complex   ☐ other vitamins:_____

   ☐ calcium   ☐ magnesium   ☐ iron   ☐ iodine

   ☐ other minerals:_____

VI. FUTURE ACTION

1. Would you be interested in learning about or sharing your knowledge of nutrition as it applies to older women?   ☐ yes   ☐ no   ☐ possibly

2. Would you be interested in participating in a discussion group, with older women, concerning health and social problems of older women?

   ☐ yes   ☐ no   ☐ possibly

   If yes, do you prefer   ☐ a small group (4 to 8)   ☐ larger group (10 to 15)

3. Would you be interested in talking about your health and/or social problems with a concerned individual?   ☐ yes   ☐ no   ☐ possibly

4. Would you be interested in learning skills to use in a menopause clinic?

   ☐ yes   ☐ no   ☐ possibly

5. Are there any subjects you would like to learn about or any topics you would like to discuss with other women? (Specify):

   _____

   _____

We welcome any comments you would care to add:

VII. ETHNIC BACKGROUND

1. Race (check more than one if applicable) ☐ a. American Indian
   ☐ b. Asian ☐ c. Black ☐ d. Caucasian ☐ e. Mexican American
   ☐ f. Other (specify): _____
2. Religion ☐ a. Buddhist ☐ b. Catholic ☐ c. Jewish ☐ d. Protestant
   (specify Protestant—) _____
   ☐ e. Other (specify): _____

VIII. CONTRACEPTIVE HISTORY

What kind of contraception, if any, are you using or have you used?

1. ☐ Pill For how long? _____
2. ☐ IUD
3. ☐ diaphragm
4. ☐ condoms
5. ☐ foam

6. ☐ rhythm
7. ☐ spermicidal creams or jelly
8. ☐ sterilization—male
   ☐ sterilization—female
9. other _____

ADDENDA: Questions we forgot to ask:

1. At what age did you notice the first of the symptoms checked in section III? _____
2. If you had a hysterectomy (II., 9), were your ovaries also removed? _____

Suggested Readings

The comments about the books are quoted from the women who recommended them. Most of the books are available in public libraries. Some of them are in paperback.

CHAPTER ONE:
WHAT GOES ON BEHIND THE SHEET?

Boston Women's Health Book Collective. *Our Bodies, Ourselves.*
New York: Simon and Schuster, 1976.
This book is strongly feminist. It contains lots of valuable information, and has a good chapter on evaluating and communicating with doctors.
Lanson, Lucienne, M.D. *From Woman To Woman.*
New York: Alfred A. Knopf, 1975.
This is the best general information I've found about women's health problems—the illustrations are especially helpful in making things clear.
Levin, Arthur, M. D. *Talk Back To Your Doctor.*
New York: Doubleday and Company, 1975.
The chapter on advice to women is very good. I'm going to ask questions the next time I see my doctor.
Notman, Malkah T. and Nadelson, Carol, eds. *The Woman As Patient.*
New York: Plenum Press, 1976.
The chapter on menopause stresses emotional aspects.
Samuel, Mike, M.D. and Bennet, Hal. *The Well Body Book.*
New York: Random House, 1973.
This takes the mystery out of doctoring.

CHAPTER TWO:
WHAT DOES MENOPAUSE MEAN?

Connell, Elizabeth B., M.D. *Hormones, Sex and Happiness.*
Chicago, Illinois: Cowles Book Company, 1971.
The doctor gives a good picture of the whole endocrine gland system and a little bit about menopause.
Kaufman, Sherwin A., M.D. *The Ageless Woman. Menopause, Hormones, and the Quest for Youth.*
Englewood Cliffs, N.J.: Prentice-Hall, Inc., 1967.
Though somewhat dated and occasionally patronizing, this book includes interesting historical and crosscultural information about menopause.
LeBaron, Ruthann. *Hormones, A Delicate Balance.*
New York: Bobbs-Merrill Company, 1972.
The author is a professor of biology, so her book is a bit technical, but this is an excellent description of the interrelationship of the endocrine glands and the nervous system.

Riedman, Sarah R. *Hormones: How They Work.*
New York: Abelard-Schuman, 1973
This is a book for young people, so it's a simple but interesting explanation of the endocrine system.

Ruebsaat, Helmut J., M.D. *The Male Climacteric.* New York: Hawthorn Books Inc., 1975.
This is a kind of "men suffer too" book. Raymond Hull writes a personal account of his symptoms in the first part, then the doctor discusses male "menopause." It's strange, if true; most doctors don't agree.

Weideger, Paula. *Menstruation and Menopause. The Physiology and Psychology, The Myth and The Reality.*
New York: Alfred A. Knopf, 1976.
Menstruation is the main interest of this book, but there is information about menopause, with the emphasis on its psychological aspects. If you can ignore the overdocumented style, you will find some unusual information.

BOOKS ON BREAST DISEASE

Kushner, Rose. *Breast Cancer. A Personal History and Investigative Report.* New York: Harcourt, Brace, Jovanovich, 1975.
A courageous and thorough study of all aspects of the disease. She pulls no punches about its incidence or the survival chances of its victims.

Lasser, Terese and Clarke, William Kendall. *Reach to Recovery.*
New York: Simon and Schuster, 1972.
This book was recommended by a friend who has had breast surgery. Terese Lasser writes about her own experience and her development of a program in which women help each other in recovery from mastectomies.

Rollin, Betty. *First, You Cry.* New York: J. B. Lippincott Company, 1976.
This television reporter, who couldn't believe it could happen to her, tells a very personal story about her surgery. Sometimes her tongue is too sharp, but she reveals important insights into her psychological reactions.

Strax, Philip, M.D. *Early Detection. Breast Cancer Is Curable.*
New York: New American Library, 1974.
Dr. Strax specializes in treatment of the disease, so he provides a good deal of medical information. But, as the title suggests, his is a hopeful approach.

CHAPTER THREE:
WHAT ABOUT HORMONE THERAPY?

We decided not to recommend any books about hormone therapy. We have not found an objective, up-to-date treatment of the subject. Watch magazines and newspapers for the latest developments.

CHAPTER FOUR:
HOW WAS HORMONE THERAPY DEVELOPED?

Atherton, Gertrude. *Black Oxen*. New York: Boni and Liveright, 1923.
This is the novel that caused a great stir in the twenties because it is about a woman who was rejuvenated with hormones. It is old-fashioned and flowery, but great fun to read.

Corners, George F. *Rejuvenation. How Steinach Makes People Young*.
New York: Thomas Seltzer, 1923
The Steinach method is the one Atherton wrote about. If you can find this book, it will provide an interesting historical perspective to hormone therapy.

Voronoff, Serge. *The Conquest of Life*. New York: Brentano's, 1928.
Like the book about Steinach, this gives an historical insight into the development of hormone therapy. But the "monkey-gland" expert himself wrote this one.

CHAPTER FIVE:
HOW DID OUR GRANDMOTHERS TREAT MENOPAUSE?

Beecher, Catharine E. *Letters to the People on Health and Happiness*.
New York: Harper and Brothers, 1855.
Reprint by Arno Press, Inc., 1972.
Since this book was reissued a few years ago, it might be available through the public library. It gives a vivid idea about conditions and attitudes toward women's health in the midnineteenth century.

Blackwell, Elizabeth, M.D. *Pioneer Work for Women*.
New York: E. P. Dutton and Company, 1914.
Dr. Blackwell's story about her struggle to become a doctor does not discuss menopause, but it shows what general attitudes toward health care were like in the nineteenth century.

Delaney, Janice, Lupton, Mary Jane, and Toth, Emily. *The Curse: A Cultural History of Menstruation*.
New York: E. P. Dutton and Company, 1976.
I haven't seen this book yet, but the reviews suggest that it gives a very long historical view of cultural attitudes toward women's "peculiar" biology. Though its emphasis is on menstruation, it must, indirectly, deal with menopause too.

Farnham, Eliza. *Woman and Her Era*. 2 vols.
New York: C. M. Pumb and Company, 1865.
It is in volume one (pp. 55-72) where this early feminist's remark able commentary about menopause appears. Her opinions certainly contradict what the doctors of her time were saying about "the change."

Gunn, John C., M.D. *Domestic Medicine, or The Poor Man's Friend in the Hours of Affliction, Pain, and Sickness*.
Philadelphia: G. V. Raymond, 1840.
If you can find this, or any old home-remedy medical book, you can relive the days of herbal tonics and blood-letting. You also realize how much people depended upon themselves for health care.

Michaelis, Karen. *The Dangerous Age.*
New York: John Lane and Company, 1911.
This Danish novel caused a sensation because it tells the story of a
middle-aged woman who left her husband and found a young
lover. It also discreetly alludes to menopause.

CHAPTER SIX:
WHAT CONDITIONS MAY REQUIRE SURGERY?

Lanson, Lucienne, M.D. *From Woman to Woman.*
New York: Alfred A. Knopf, 1975.
We mention Dr. Lanson's book again here because it includes the
clearest discussion we have found about conditions which may lead
to hysterectomies.
Nugent, Nancy. *Hysterectomy: A Complete Up-To-Date Guide To
Everything About It and Why It May Be Needed.*
Garden City, N.Y.: Doubleday and Company, 1976.
The medical information is a bit sketchy, but she has included some
revealing personal interviews with women about their varied
experiences and reactions.

CHAPTER SEVEN:
WHAT HAPPENS TO SEXUALITY?

Blankenship,Judy, ed. *Scenes from Life: Views of Marriage, Family, and
Intimacy.* Boston: Little, Brown and Company, 1976.
This book has articles on women of all ages; it is especially good on
women alone.
Brothers, Joyce, Ph.D. *Better Than Ever.*
New York: Simon and Schuster, 1975.
I didn't like a lot of the book. There's too much emphasis on
keeping thin and beautiful. But the chapters on sex are something
else, especially the one which advocates extramarital affairs for
women as a way of keeping a marriage lively. She adds, though,
that such activity is much too stressful for middle-aged men.
Comfort, Alex, Ph.D. *The Joy of Sex.*
New York: Simon and Schuster, 1972
Very explicit, but it does suggest ways to relax and enjoy sex.
Cox, Sue. *Female Psychology: The Emerging Self.*
Chicago: Science Research Associates, 1976.
I recommend this book because it offers information about cultural
and ethnic differences toward sexuality and other aspects of female
behavior, as well as specific ideas about how women can better
understand themselves.
Felstein, Ivor, M.D. *Sex in Later Life.* Baltimore: Penguin Books, 1973.
Dr. Felstein comes across as a charming British doctor, offering a
low-key discussion of many aspects of sex in later years.

Kaplan, Helen Singer. *The New Sex Therapy.*
New York: New York Times Book Company, 1974.
A sex therapist recommended this to me as a comprehensive
treatment of the subject (with a good bibliography), but it is also
a kind of how-to-do-it book too.

Katchadourian, Herant A., M.D. *Human Sexuality. Sense and Nonsense.*
San Francisco: Freeman, 1974.
This is a sensible discussion of many varieties of sexual experience.

Masters, W. H., M.D. and Virginia E. Johnson. *Human Sexual Response.*
Boston: Little, Brown and Company, 1966.
Surely everybody knows about Masters and Johnson and their
pioneering work in sexuality. This is a readable discussion based
on their original work.

Masters, W. H., M.D. and Virginia E. Johnson. *The Pleasure Bond.*
Boston: Little, Brown, and Company, 1974.
This later book by the sex experts is especially interesting because
it consists of transcriptions of discussions among groups of their
patients about their sexual adjustments and experiences.

CHAPTER EIGHT:
WHAT ABOUT LIFE'S OTHER CHANGES?

DeRosis, Helen, M.D. and Pellegrino, Victoria Y. *The Book of Hope.*
New York: Macmillan Company, 1976.
I think this book will be especially helpful because it not only
discusses depression among women of all ages, but gives specific
suggestions as to how it can be overcome. I like the emphasis on
physical activity.

Harris, Janet. *Prime of Ms. America.* New York: G. P. Putnam's Sons, 1975.
A newly divorced friend of mine recommended this book to me;
she thought it was especially good on advice to women alone.

Huyck, Margaret Hellie. *Growing Older.*
Englewood Cliffs, N.J.: Prentice-Hall, Inc., 1974.
It's worthwhile to wade through the social-science language because
of the several provocative writers who are quoted.

Janeway, Elizabeth. *Between Myth and Morning.*
New York: William Morrow Company, 1975.
Janeway speaks so well for middle-aged women. This is a good
introduction to her work. It is based on several articles she has
written at different times.

Janeway, Elizabeth. *Man's World, Woman's Place.*
New York: Dell Publishers, 1972.
This is the best book I've read about how women feel about
themselves and how they got that way.

Lessing, Doris. *The Summer Before the Dark.* New York: Alfred Knopf, 1973.
Whether you will like this novel about a middle-aged woman, the
eternal nurturer, will depend on how you feel about yourself, I guess.

Neugarten, Bernice L., ed. *Middle Age and Aging.*
Chicago: University of Chicago Press, 1968.
This is a textbook about many aspects of aging, but the chapter by
Neugarten about women's attitudes concerning menopause is
especially appropriate.
Sheehy, Gail. *Passages. Predictable Crises of Adult Life.*
New York: E. P. Dutton and Company, 1976.
This deals with women of all ages, so it should help to put things
into perspective for all of us.

CHAPTER NINE:
WHAT CAN WOMEN DO FOR THEMSELVES?

EXERCISE

Cooper, Mildred and Kenneth H., M.D. *Aerobics for Women.*
New York: M. Evans and Company, 1972.
I like this book because it gives instructions for strenuous exercises
to develop heart and lungs.
Ellfeldt, Lois, Ph.D. and Lowman, Charles L., M.D. *Exercises for the
Mature Adult.* Springfield, Illinois: Charles C. Thomas, 1973.
These authors give a lot of medical information about the structure
of the body and what each exercise does to strengthen the muscles.
Feldenkrais, Moshe. *Awareness Through Movement.*
New York: Harper and Row, 1972.
A friend told me that this man's techniques of muscle manipulation
had improved her whole life. With a recommendation like that, it
would probably be well worth it to study this rather difficult book.
Mensendieck, Bess M., M.D. *Look Better, Feel Better.*
New York: Harper and Brothers, 1954.
I learned these simple exercises way back when I was in college and
they have helped me ever since.
Royal Canadian Air Force Exercise Plans for Physical Fitness.
New York: Pocket Books, Inc., 1962.
My doctor recommended this book because the exercises are geared
to different ages and abilities.
Rush, Anne Kent. *Getting Clear. Body Work for Women.*
New York: Random House, 1973.
Anne Rush's "body work" involves much more than exercises; she
shows you how to think about your body in a different way.

Books on Yoga

There seem to be hundreds of different books on yoga, but these three
have been recommended as giving clear and simple directions without
too much on the philosophy:

Devi, Indra. *Yoga for Americans.* New York: Signet, 1968.
Phelan, Nancy and Volin, Michael. *Yoga Over Forty.*
New York: Harper and Row, 1965.

Zorn, William. *Body Harmony: The Easy Yoga Exercise Way.*
New York: Hawthorn Books, Inc., 1971.

Books on Relaxation Techniques

Benson, Herbert, M.D. *The Relaxation Response.*
New York: William Morrow and Company, Inc., 1975.
Dr. Benson describes just what happens to your body when you
relax, and he gives specific directions on how to do it.
Hemingway, Patricia Drake. *The Transcendental Meditation Primer.*
New York: David McKay Company, Inc., 1975.
The author describes TM's techniques and results clearly and
persuasively. She helps you understand why so many Americans
are doing it.

EAT WELL

Adams, Catherine F. *Nutritive Value of American Foods.*
Washington, D.C.: United States Department of Agriculture, 1975.
This is a very comprehensive list of foods, their nutritive value, and
calories.
Deutsh, Ronald M. *The Family Guide to Better Food and Better Health.*
Des Moines, Iowa: Creative Home Library, 1971.
A public librarian recommended this book as being one of the most
comprehensive and popular sources of information about nutrition.
Lappe, Frances Moore. *Diet for a Small Planet.*
New York: Ballantine Books, 1972.
The author explains why it's wise to become a vegetarian, and she's
pretty convincing.
Robinson, Corinne. *Basic Nutrition and Diet Therapy.*
New York: Macmillan and Company, 1970.
This is a textbook for nurses, but it is full of information about
nutrition that we can all use.
Stuart, Robert B. and Davis, Barbara. *Slim Chance in a Fat World.*
Guilford, Ct.: Dushkin Publishing Company, 1972.
This book tells how to use behavior modification to lose weight. It has
very specific suggestions, many of which have helped me lose a few
pounds.
Taylor, Renee. *Hunza Health Secrets for Long Life and Happiness.*
Englewood Cliffs, N.J.: Prentice-Hall, 1967.
A doctor who believes that diet is the key to good health recom-
mended this book to me. The Hunza people are famous for their
good health and longevity.
Williams, Roger, *Nutrition Against Disease.* New York: Bantam, 1972.
The author is a specialist in nutrition who makes this complicated
subject very clear.

Williams, Roger. *Nutrition in a Nutshell.* New York: Dolphin Books, 1962.
This is an early book by the same food expert, but it's still a good
source of information about diet.

TALK TOGETHER

Alberti, Robert E. and Emmons, Michael L. *Your Perfect Right: A Guide to
Assertive Behavior.* San Luis Obispo, California: Impact Books, 1970.
This is a comprehensive study of assertiveness training which is often
used as a textbook.
Berne, Eric. *Games People Play.* New York: Grove Press, 1964.
This is a good introduction to the concepts of Transactional Analysis.
Berne, Eric. *What Do You Say After You Say Hello?*
New York: Grove Press, 1972.
Berne develops his ideas about Transactional Analysis more fully in
this later book.
Faraday, Ann. *The Dream Game.* New York: Harper and Row, 1974.
The author, who is a specialist in dreams, shows how a person can use
her dreams to understand herself better.
Faraday, Ann. *Dream Power.* New York: Berkley Publishing Corp., 1973.
This is an earlier book in which the author introduces her theories
about the importance of dreams.
First Assertive Rap Group of Seattle-King County NOW. *Woman Assert
Yourself.* New York: Harper and Row, 1976.
The women who participated in a rap group show how they learned
the techniques of assertiveness training, through transcriptions of
some of their sessions.
James, Muriel and Jongewald, Dorothy. *Born to Win: Transactional Analysis
with Gestalt Experiments.*
Reading, Mass.: Addison-Wesley Publishing Company, 1971.
This is an extension of Eric Berne's work. It includes specific exercises.
Perls, Frederick S. *Gestalt Therapy Verbatim.*
Moab, Utah: Real People Press, 1969.
This book consists of transcriptions of Gestalt therapy sessions. It is
an interesting way to learn about its concepts and techniques.
Simon, Sidney B., Howe, Leland W., and Kirschenbaum, Howard. *Values
Clarification.* New York: Hart Publishing Company, 1972.
This book helps a person decide what her values are and shows her
how to make choices.
Steiner, Claude. *Scripts People Live.* New York: Grove Press, 1974.
Steiner is a disciple of Eric Berne. In this book he shows how people
are conditioned to behave the way they do.

Glossary

These definitions are intended to help the reader talk with medical personnel and read technical information more easily. A key to pronunciation is supplied with those words that seem especially difficult.

a-, an- Prefix meaning not, without.

adrenal gland One of a pair of ductless glands located above the kidneys.

amenorrhea (a-men-o-re'ah) Absence of the menses.

androgen Any of various hormones that control the appearance and development of masculine characteristics, as testosterone and androsterone.

anovulation Suspension or cessation of ovulation.

arteriosclerosis Hardening of the arteries.

aspirator An apparatus for removing fluid by suction from any of the body cavities.

biopsy The process of removing tissue from living patients for diagnosis.

carcinogenic Causing cancer.

carcinoma Cancer.

cardiovascular Relating to the heart and the blood vessels or the circulation

-cele A suffix denoting a swelling or hernia.

cervix The neck or mouth of the uterus.

climacteric (kli-mak'ter-ik, kli-mak-ter'ik) A period of life occurring in women preceding termination of the reproductive period.

clitoris (kli'to-ris, klit'o-ris) A small erectile organ at the upper part of the vulva.

coitus (ko'i-tus) Sexual intercourse.

contraindicate To indicate the danger or undesirability of a drug or treatment.

corpus luteum The yellow endocrine body formed in the ovary in the site of a ruptured ovarian follicle.

curettage (ku-rah-tazh') A scraping of the interior of a cavity for the removal of abnormal tissue or to obtain material for tissue diagnosis.

cyst An abnormal sac containing gas, fluid, or a semisolid material.

cystic mastitis A benign disease of the breast.

cystocele Hernia of the bladder.

D and C Dilatation and Curettage A minor surgical procedure in which the cervical canal is enlarged to permit the scraping of the interior of the uterus.

diuretic A medication which increases the excretion of urine.

dys- Prefix meaning bad or difficult.

dysmenorrhea (dis-men-o-re'ah) Difficult and painful menstruation.

dyspareunia (dis-pa-ru'ni-ah) Pain during sexual intercourse.

dysuria Difficulty or pain in urination.

ERT Estrogen replacement therapy.

-ectomy Suffix meaning the removal of any organ or gland.

edema (e-de'ma) Abnormal accumulation of fluid within the body tissues which produces swelling.

endocrine gland One of several ductless glands which secrete hormones directly into the bloodstream and which have a critical importance in many phases of physiological activity.

endogenous (en-doj'e-nus) Originating or produced within the organism or one of its parts, as endogenous estrogen.

endometrial (en-do-me'tri-al) Relating to the inner lining of the uterine wall.

endometriosis (en-do-me-tri-o'sis) A pelvic condition in which fragments of endometrial tissue are found outside the confines of the uterine cavity.

endometrium (en-do-me'tri-um) The mucous membrane comprising the inner layer of the uterine wall.

estrogen Any of various hormones that control the appearance and development of feminine characteristics, as estradiol, estriol, and estrone.

exogenous (eks-oj'e-nus) Originating or produced outside the organism, as exogenous estrogen.

Fallopian tube One of two tubes which branch from either side of the uterus; the tube through which the ovum passes from the ovary to the uterus.

fibrocystic disease of the breast A nonmalignant breast condition characterized by multiple small cysts and fibrous thickening of the breast tissue.

fibroid A nonmalignant tumor involving the wall of the uterus; also called leiomyomas or myomas.

follicle One of the numerous sacs in the ovary containing an ovum; sometimes called Graafian follicle.

follicle stimulating hormone (FSH) Pituitary hormone which stimulates the growth and development of ovarian follicles.

genitalia Sexual organs; the organs of reproduction.

gonad An organ which produces sex cells; the testis of the male and the ovary of the female.

gonadotropin (gon-a-do-tro'pin) A hormone capable of promoting gonadal growth and function, such as the pituitary hormones FSH and LH.

hemorrhage Excessively heavy bleeding, either internal or external.

hirsuitism Abnormal presence of excessive facial and/or body hair, especially in women.

hormone A chemical substance formed in one organ or part of the body and carried in the blood to another organ or part, usually produced by an endocrine gland.

hyperplasia An increase in number of cells in a tissue or organ whereby the bulk of the part or organ is increased; often refers to build-up of endometrial tissue.

hypertension High blood pressure.

hypomenorrhea A lessening of the flow or a shortening of the duration of menstruation.

hypothalamus A control center at the base of the brain which regulates body temperature, many metabolic processes, and certain emotional states.

hysterectomy Surgical removal of the uterus and cervix either by an abdominal incision or through the vagina.

introitus (in-tro'i-tus) The entrance to the vagina.

-itis Suffix meaning inflammation of, as in vaginitis.

labia The lip-like folds of the vulva; labia majora, the outer lips and labia minora, the inner lips.

lesion Any unusual or abnormal change in the structure of an organ or tissue.

luteinizing hormone (LH) Pituitary hormone which stimulates ovulation and the production of progesterone.

malignant Cancerous.

mammography X-ray of the breasts for the detection of abnormal tissue change.

mast-, masto- Combining forms meaning breast.

mastectomy Surgical removal of the breast.

mastitis Inflammation of the breast.

maturation index A method for determining estrogen levels by analysis of the types of cells in vaginal tissue.

menopause The cessation of menses.

menorrhagia (men-o-ra′ji-ah) Excessively profuse or prolonged menstruation.

menses Menstrual flow.

menstrual cycle The time interval from the beginning of one menstrual period to the beginning of the next.

metabolism The sum of the chemical changes whereby the function of nutrition is carried out.

metrorrhagia (me-tro-ra′ji-ah) Bleeding from the uterus between periods.

myoma Fibroid tumor of the uterus.

myomectomy Surgical removal of a myoma.

neoplasm Any abnormal growth of tissue in the body.

nocturia Urinating at night.

-oma Suffix meaning tumor, as in fibroma, meaning a tumor composed of fibrous tissue.

oophorectomy (o-of′or-ek′to-me) Surgical removal of an ovary.

orgasm The physical sensation of sexual release at the climax of coitus, masturbation, or other sexual play.

osteoporosis (os-te-o-po-ro′sis) Reduction in the quantity of bone, leading to its general weakening.

ovary The female sex gland.

ovulation The release of an ovum from the ovarian follicle.

ovum, plural **ova** The female sex cell produced by the ovaries.

palpate To examine by feeling and pressing with the palms of the hands and fingers.

Pap smear Common name for Papanicolaou smear. A method whereby cells from the vagina are microscopically examined for any abnormal changes. Used as a screening method for cervical cancer.

parathyroid gland One of several small glands found near the thyroid gland.

perimenopausal During the menopause.

perineum The area between the vagina and the rectum.

pituitary gland One of the endocrine glands, located at the base of the brain.

polyp A membrane growth, usually nonmalignant, that grows on a stalk; cervical and endometrial polyps are not uncommon.

postmenopausal After the menopause.

premenopausal Before the menopause.

progesterone The ovarian hormone produced by the corpus luteum as a result of ovulation.

progestin Any substance that produces the biological changes of progesterone; sometimes termed progestogen.

prolapse A falling down of an organ because of inadequate muscular support, as in a prolapsed uterus.

pubococcygeus muscle (pu-bo-kok-sij'e-us) A band muscle which stretches between the pubic bone in front to the coccyx (tail bone) in back and helps to support the female pelvic organs.

rectocele A bulging of the rectal wall into the vaginal canal.

salpingectomy Surgical removal of a Fallopian tube.

salpingitis Inflammation of the Fallopian tubes.

salpingo- Combining form meaning tube, usually refers to the Fallopian tubes.

speculum An instrument that enlarges a passageway for the purpose of inspecting the interior, as the vagina and cervix.

testosterone The male sex hormone responsible for male sexual characteristics.

thermography A diagnostic procedure to detect cancerous breast tumors by measuring temperature differences within breast tissue.

thromboembolism The blockage of a blood vessel by a blood clot or other material.

thyroid gland One of the endocrine glands, located near the windpipe.

urethra The passageway leading from the urinary bladder to the outside.

urethrocele A bulging of the urethral wall into the vaginal canal.

uterus The womb; the hollow muscular organ in which the impregnated ovum is developed into the child.

vagina The birth canal, extending from the uterus to the outside.

vaginitis Any inflammation or infection of the vagina.

vasomotor Causing dilation or constriction of the blood vessels.

vulva The external genitalia of the female.

vulvitis Inflammation of the vulva.

REFERENCES

Adams, Catherine F. *Nutritive Value of American Foods.* Agriculture
Handbook No. 456. Washington, D.C.: United States Department
of Agriculture, 1975.

Atherton, Gertrude. *Adventures of a Novelist.*
New York: Liveright, Inc., 1932.

Atkinson, Caroline B., ed. *Letters of Susan Hale.*
Boston: Marshall Jones Co., 1918.

Bart, Pauline. "The Loneliness of the Long-Distance Mother."
In *Women: A Feminist Perspective*, ed. by Jo Freeman.
PaloAlto, California: Mayfield Publishing Company, 1975.

Beecher, Catharine. *Letters to the People on Health and Happiness.*
New York: Harper and Row, 1855.
Reprint. New York:
Arno Press, 1972.

Benjamin, Harry J. "The Story of Rejuvenation." *American Mercury*,
December 1935, pp. 480-483.

Bishop, Jerry E. "Studies Hint at Link of Uterine Cancer, Menopause
Therapy." *The Wall Street Journal*, 4 December 1975.

Blackwell, Elizabeth. *Pioneer Work for Women.*
New York: E. P. Dutton and Company, 1914.

Bohlinder, Clorinda S. S. and Greenblatt, Robert B. "The Patho-
physiology of the Hot Flush," In *The Menopausal Syndrome*, ed. by
Robert B. Greenblatt, M.D., Virenda B. Mahesh, Ph.D., Paul G.
McDonough, M.D. New York: Medcom Press, 1974.

Burton, Jean. *Lydia Pinkham Is Her Name.*
New York: Farrar, Strauss, and Company, 1949.

Clarke, Edward H., M.D. *Sex in Education; or A Fair Chance for Girls.*
Boston: James R. Osgood and Company, 1875.

Corners, George F. *Rejuvenation. How Steinach Makes People Young.*
New York: Thomas Seltzer, 1923.

"Cures for Old Age." *The Literary Digest*, 21 September 1929, p. 22.

Curtis, Lindsay, M.D. "For Women Only." *The Seattle Times*,
7 December 1975.

Davis, M. Edward, M.D. *A Doctor Discusses Menopause and Estrogens.*
New York: Budlong Press Company, 1969.

De L'Isere, Colombat. *A Treatise on the Diseases and Special Hygiene of
Females.* Translated by Charles D. Meigs, M.D.

Dixon, Edward H., M.D. *Woman and Her Diseases From the Cradle to the
Grave.* 5th rev. ed. New York: Charles H. Ring, 1847.

Farnham, Eliza W. *Woman and Her Era.* 2 vols.
New York: C. M. Plumb and Company, 1865.

Ferin, Jacques, et al. "Ovarian Conservation Versus Extirpation:
A Panel." In *The Menopausal Syndrome*, ed. by Robert B. Greenblatt,
M.D., Virenda B. Mahesh, Ph.D., Paul G. McDonough, M.D.

Food. The Yearbook of Agriculture 1959.
Washington, D.C.: United States Department of Agriculture, 1959.

Frank, Robert T., M.D. *The Female Sex Hormone.*
London: Bailliere, Tindall and Cox, 1929.

Frank, Robert T., M.D. "A Review of the Progress in Endocrinology of
Interest to the Gynecologist and Obstetrician." *American Journal of
Obstetrics and Gynecology 20* (August 1930): 215-220

Geist, Samuel H., M.D. "Are Estrogens Carcinogenic in the Human
Female?" *American Journal of Obstetrics and Gynecology* 42
(August 1941): 242-248
Geist, Samuel H., M.D. and Spielman, Frank, M.D. "Therapeutic Value
of Theelin in Menopause." *American Journal of Obstetrics and
Gynecology* 23 (January-June 1932): 701.
Gunn, John C., M.D. *Domestic Medicine or the Poor Man's Friend in the
Hours of Affliction, Pain, and Sickness.*
Philadelphia: G. V. Raymond, 1840.
Gusberg, S. B., M.D. "Precursors of Corpus Carcinoma Estrogens and
Adenomatous Hyperplasia." *American Journal of Obstetrics and
Gynecology 54* (December 1947): 905-925.
Hathaway, M. L. and Foard, E. D. *Heights and Weights of Adults in the
United States.* Home Economics Research Report No. 10.
Washington, D.C.: United States Department of Agriculture, 1960.
Hoover, Robert, M.D., et al. "Menopausal Estrogen and Breast Cancer."
The New England Journal of Medicine 295 (9 August 1976): 401-405.
"Hope for Grandmothers." *NewsweekMagazine,* 28 June 1954, p. 82.
"Hormone Profits." *Business Week,* 11 September 1943, pp. 70-71.
"Hormones for Depression." *Newsweek Magazine,* 6 January 1975, p. 56.
Jern, Helen Z., M.D. *Hormone Therapy of the Menopause and Aging.*
Springfield, Illinois: Charles C. Thomas, 1973.
Kegel, Arnold H., M.D. "Physiologic Therapy of Urinary Stress
Incontinence." *Monographs on Surgery* (1952): 120-129.
Kisch, E. Heinrich, M.D. *The Sexual Life of Women in Its Physiological,
Pathological and Hygienic Ascpects.* Translated by M. Eden Paul, M.D.
New York: Rebman and Company, 1910.
Leyda, Jay. *The Years and Hours of Emily Dickinson.* 2 vols.
New Haven, Ct.: Yale University Press, 1960.
Lincoln, Miriam, *You'll Live Through It.*
New York: Harper Brothers, 1961.
Mack, Thomas, et al. "Estrogens and Endometrial Cancer in a Retire-
ment Community." *The New England Journal of Medicine* 294 (3 June
1976): 1262-1267.
Mead, Margaret. *Male and Female.*
New York: William Morrow and Company, 1949.
Meigs, Charles D., M.D. *Woman: Her Diseases and Remedies. Letters to His
Class.* 3rd rev. ed. Philadelphia: Blanchard and Lea, 1854.
Mendelsohn, Robert, M.D. "To Your Health." *Seattle Post-Intelligencer,*
24 June 1976.
Menopause. Los Angeles: Professional Research, Inc., 1971.
Menopause and Aging. DHEW Publication No. 73-319.
Washington, D.C.: Department of Health, Education
and Welfare, 1971.
"Menopause Weakens the Heart." *The Seattle Times,* 24 November 1975.
Michaelis, Karin. *The Dangerous Age.*
New York: John Lane Company, 1911.
Morris, Ruby Weitzer. *Cultural Attitudes Toward the Menopause Among a
Non-Western Group of Women.* Master's Thesis, University of
Washington, 1960.

163

Myths of Vitamins. DHEW Publication No. 76-2047.
Washington, D.C.: Department of Health, Education and
Welfare, 1976.

Novak, Emil, M.D. "An Appraisal of Ovarian Therapy," *Endocrinology*
6 (September 1922): 599-620.

Novak, Emil, M.D. and Y ui, Enmei, M.D. "Relation of Endometrial
Hyperplasia to Adenocarcinoma of the Uterus." *American Journal
of Obstetrics and Gynecology* 32 (1936): 674-695.

" 'Over-Reaction' to Estrogen-Ca Link Seen Detrimental," *Medical
Tribune,* 7 July 1976.

Page, L. and Fincher, L. J. *Food and Your Weight.* Home and Garden
Bulletin No. 74. Washington, D.C.: United States Department of
Agriculture, 1964.

Recommended Dietary Allowances. 8th rev. ed. Food and Nutrition Board,
National Research Council. Washingtonm, D.C.: National Academy
of Sciences, 1974.

Reuben, David, M.D. *Everything Your Always Wanted to Know About Sex
But Were Afraid To Ask.* New York: D. McKay, 1969.

Rodgers, Joann. "Rush to Surgery." *New York Times Magazine,*
21 September 1975.

Ryan, Kenneth. J., M.D. "Cancer Risk and Estrogen Use in the
Menopause." *The New England Journal of Medicine* 293 (4 December
1975): 1199-1200.

"Sex Hormones in Legal Battle." *Business Week,* 22 December 1945, p. 46.

Smith, Donald C., M.D. et al. "Association of Exogenous Estrogen and
Endometrial Carcinoma." *The New England Journal of Medicine* 293
(4 December 1975): 1164-1167.

Smith-Rosenberg, Carroll. "Puberty to Menopause: The Cycle of
Femininity in Nineteenth Century America." In *Clio's Conscious-
ness Raised,* ed. by Mary Hartman and Lois W. Banner.
New York: Harper and Brothers, 1974.

Stedman's Medical Dictionary. 23rd ed.
Baltimore: The Williams and Wilkins Company, 1976.

Strongin, Herman F. "Woman — Her Critical Decade: A Warning
and a Plea." *American Medicine* (November 1933): 536.

Van de Water, Virginia. "Ordeals of the Middle-Aged Woman."
Good Housekeeping Magazine, July 1912, pp. 91-94.

Voronoff, Serge. *The Conquest of Life.* Translated by G. Gibier
Rambaud, M.D. New York: Brentano's, 1928.

Weiss, Noel, S., M.D. "Increasing Incidence of Endometrial Cancer in
the United States." *The New England Journal of Medicine* 294
(3 July 1976): 1259-1262.

Weiss, Noel S., M.D. "Risks and Benefits of Estrogen Use." *The New
England Journal of Medicine* 293 (4 December 1975): 1200-1201.

Wilson, Robert A., M.D. *Feminine Forever.*
New York: M. Evans and Company, 1966.

Wright, Ralph C., M.D. "Hysterectomy: Past, Present, and Future."
Obstetrics and Gynecology (April 1969): 560-563.

Ziel, Harry K., M.D. and Finkle, William D., Ph.D. "Increased Risk of
Endometrial Carcinoma Among Users of Conjugated Estrogens."
The New England Journal of Medicine 293 (4 December 1975):1167-1170.

INDEX

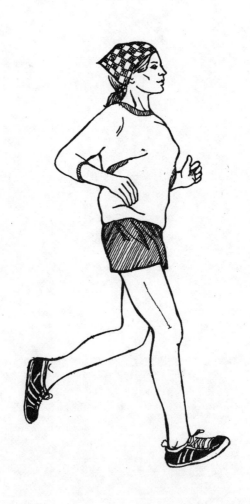